INTRODUCTION TO MALARIA PROBLEM IN INDIA

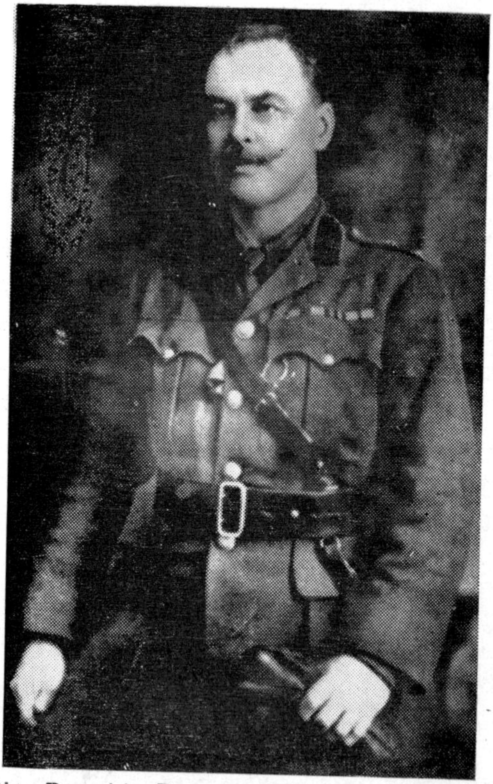

Sir Ronald Ross (1857-1932). Indian Medical Services 1881-1899; later Professor of Tropical Sanitation University of Liverpool and Liverpool School of Tropical Medicine; Physician for Tropical Diseases Kings College Hospital London Director-in-Chief Ross Institute and Hospital for Tropital Diseases London.

Demostrated malaria parasites in the mosquito that had fed on blood of malaria patient on August 20, 1897, at Secunderabad; completed the life cycle of the malaria parasite on July 9, 1898 supplied proof of malaria transmission by mosquito. Awarded in 1902, Nobel Prize for Physiology and Medicine.

INTRODUCTION TO MALARIA PROBLEM IN INDIA

Vedic Period to Early 1950s

The Dosabhai Hormasji Cama Prize Essay 1944, University of Bombay

B. L. RAINA

With an Introduction by

Dr. Jivraj N. Mehta
M.D. (London), M.R.C.P. (London)

Commonwealth Publishers
NEW DELHI-110002
(INDIA)

Also by B.L. Raina

***Planning Family in India Pre-Vedic to Early 1950s**

***Social Situation in India**

***Population Policy**

***Health Science in Ancient India**

***Health Science March Through Centuries**

***The Quest for a Small Family**

***World War II—Medical Services of India**

First Edition : 1951

Second Edition : 1991

ISBN 81-7169-108-0

Published by :
Commonwealth Publishers
4378/4B, Ansari Road, Gali Murari Lal
New Delhi-110002

Printed at :
Stylish Composing Agency
Bhajanpura, Delhi-110053

ACKNOWLEDGEMENTS

For the preparation of Dosabhai Hormasji Cama Prize Essay 1944 and its subsequent publication in book-form in 1951, I reiterate my gratitude to all those whose observations have been included in this book, both who have been cited in references and others ; and my indebtness to Dr. Jivraj Mehta ; University of Bombay ; Director Medical Services Army in India ; Lt. Colonel Jaswant Singh ; Dr. Biswas ; Major General Sir Gordon Covell ; Dr. A.S. Erulker ; Dr. P.M. Mehta ; Dr. Baini Prasad ; Dr. G. Ramsay ; Sir Malcolm Watson, Public Health Commissioner with the Government of India ; Directors of Malaria Institute of India, the Imperial Agriculture Institute, School of Tropical Medicine Calcutta, Public Health of Bihar, Bombay, Central Provinces and Berar, Madras, Punjab,* North West Frontier Province* and Sindh ;* Malariologist Province of Sind* ; Malaria Officer Nawapara ; Department of Health Government of India, and the Principal Jamnibhushan Ashtanga Ayurveda Vidyalaya, Calcutta ; Dr. Bisheshwar Prasad ; Saraswati Raina and Ross Institute of Tropical Hygiene London.

For this edition, special thanks are due to Saraswati, Asoka, Neera Raina, and Om and Sudha Kaul for assistance in a number of ways.

I also take this opportunity to express my gratitude to the malaria control team especially Mr. Kher Singh and all those who assisted or gave encouragement (British, Indians, Irish, Italians) in the discovery of the larvivorous fish in Yol *Schizothorax progastus* and for experiments on in bio-environmental measures in Yol.

---

*Pre-partition.

The information compiled by Mr. V.N. Rao, the Anti-malaria Assistant and sent to me by Lt. Colonel K.S. Pillai, AMC, Senior Executive Medical Officer Military Hospital Yol Camp, giving the progress of bio-environmental measures as in October 1949 (over 5 years after they were introduced) is also gratefully acknowledged.

January 1991 **B.L. Ruina**

PREFACE TO THE SECOND EDITION

The statement on malaria in *the First Five Year Plan* (1951-56) reads: "...It has been estimated that about a million deaths are caused in India every year by malaria among the 100 million people who suffer from the disease. The economic loss is estimated at several hundred crores of rupees every year. Vast fertile areas remain fallow and natural resources remain unexploited largely due to ravages of malaria. Aggregation of labour in irrigation, hydro-electric and industrial projects is attended with severe outbreaks of malaria if special measures are not taken for its control".

In 1951, when the first edition of this book was published, there were great hopes of controlling the menace of malaria. These expectations were reinforced by the successful control of malaria during the World War II in the Eastern Theatre* and discoveries towards the end of war of insecticides like DDT and BHC, anti-malarial drugs like paludrine, chloroquine, camoquin and primaquin and greater understanding of the malaria carrying mosquitoes. The achievements of the National Malaria Control Programme (April 1953-March 1958) gave confidence in the ability to eradicate malaria in a foreseeable future, and the National Malaria Eradication Programme was launched in April 1958.

The results of "the eradication programme", for some years, were spectacular. The National Malaria Control

*Afridi, M.K., "Malaria Control" in Raina, B.L. ed. *Preventive Medicine (Nutrition Malaria Control and Prevention of Diseases).* Combined Interservices Historical Section India and Pakistan, Ministry of Defence Government of India, New Delhi, 1961.

Programme/National Malaria Eradication Programme substantially changed the situation. The number of positive cases of malaria in India reported in 1961 was 49,151 and no death due to malaria was reported during that year.

The reports of malaria incidence from 1965 onwards gave serious jolt to the hope of early malaria eradication. The number of positive cases of malaria in India reported in 1976 were 6,467,215 and deaths 59. Several factors have been identified for the set-back—organisational, managerial, logistical, financial besides the resistance in some areas of *P. falciparum* to chloroquine and also the resistance of some malaria carrying mosquitoes to insecticides. This has led to changes in malaria control strategy. The results of modified strategy has revived hopes. The positive cases of malaria in India in 1987 (provisional) reported are 1,663,284 and deaths 185.

Malaria problem has not yet lost its sting. This has prompted the issue of the second edition of this book, as some of its parts may be of interest even at present.

For the second edition of this book I had two alternatives *viz.*: (*a*) to bring the book up-to-date ; or (*b*) to keep the text of the first edition of the book unaltered and add footnotes for up-dating information on a few selected subjects.

During June 1941—early September 1945, I was deeply engaged in public health problems including bio-environmental control of malaria in Yol, and in that period discovered a new indigenous larvivorous fish *Schizothorax progastus*.* The experience in Yol provided the background for the preparation of the First Edition. I was fully occupied, during May 1946—September 1952, with the preparation of the medical history of the Indian Armed Forces in World War II. I was also assigned the duties concerned with the Geneva Conventions of August

*Raina, B.L., *Indian Medical Gazette*, V. LXXX 5, p. 273, 1945.

12, 1949.* Since September 1956, I am involved in population activities. In between these periods I was commanding a Field Ambulance, hospitals in Khyber Pass and Kashmir and working as President of Special Medical Board. In other words, I left active field work in malaria, a very long time back. The revision of the book or writing an upto-date book on malaria in India should be done by some one currently or recently working in the public health field, preferably in malaria field. I have therefore adopted the second alternative.

The original texts has been retained. Footnotes have been added in some places to update information on selected subjects. Some parts have been omitted. Photograph of Sir Ronald Ross and some appendices, mainly relating to bio-environment, have been added.

The book gives glimpses of history of malaria, the life cycle of each of the four species of malaria parasites, the bio-nomics of the most important mosquito victors of Bangladesh, India and Pakistan, and some epidemiological features of malaria in the Indian sub-continent, anti-larval and anti-mosquito measures, bio-environmental control of malaria, chemotherapy, malaria survey and campaign some reflections on the progress made, mainly upto the early 1950s.**

* The four conventions [Geneva Convention : for the Amelioration of the Conditions of the Wounded and Sick in Armed Forces in the Field ; for the Amelioration of the conditions of this Wounded, Sick and Shipwrecked Members of the Armed Forces at Sea ; relative to the Treatment of Prisoners of War ; and relative to the Protection of Civilian Persons in Time of War] were ratified by the President of India, Dr. Rajendra Prasad on October 16, 1950.

**For concise account of recent developments refer to Narasimham, M.V.V.L. *National Malaria Eradication Programme.* National Institute of Health and Family Welfare. New Delhi, 1988. (National Health Programme Series 4, Series Editors Gupta, J.P. and Bhatnagar, S.).

The appendices include :

(*i*) Extracts relating to malaria from Health Survey and Development Committee (Bhore Committee) Report ;

(*ii*) A note on Malaria in Ancient India ;

(*iii*) Some reminiscences of Bio-Environmental Control of malaria in Yol (Kangra Valley) ;

(*iv*) Observations of Director Public Health Punjab. Dr. Butt in his note on malaria in Punjab (pre-partition) dated 17.7.1944, including on method followed for malaria forecast ;

(*v*) Extracts from circulars issued by Director Public Health Central Provinces and Berar Lt. Colonel S. N. Makand on Anti-malaria measures in 19 7, control of mosquito breeding by herbiage packing 1938, and oil booms in 1939 ;

(*vi*) Extracts from report of Malariologist Government of Sind (pre-partition) Dr. Ajwani on Malaria in Sindh including observations on malaria and construction of Llyod Barrage and canal constructions ; and

(*vii*) Observations of malaria officer Nawapara Dr. K.N. Shukla, including on Zoo-prophylaxis and other malaria control measures in 1944.

I will consider the efforts in preparing the Second edition of the book worthwhile if it contributes, even among a few readers, to a greater understanding of the malaria problem in India. I also hope that the book encourages some researchers to compile a comprehensive history of malaria in India.

New Delhi
January 1991

B. L. Raina

PREFACE TO THE FIRST EDITION

Life is a fight both within and without the body. Many death rolls are our own creations. Death is inevitable and the law of nature inexorable, but nevertheless many deaths can be postponed and lives can be prolonged by conforming to simple rules of common sense. Of all the various health problems of India malaria is one of the most important. Every minute about two persons die and four hundred suffer from malaria, and yet how many people seriously attempt to bestow their attention on it in the measure it deserves? If India is to advance in economic, agricultural and industrial fields and is to raise the earning capacity and standard of living of its inhabitants, it is essential first to improve the standard of health.

Malaria has contributed, in not a small measure, to the physical, and intellectual degeneration of many nations. The malaria-carrying mosquito, which has reduced colonies of human population to a few disease-stricken individuals, has surrendered unconditionally when confronted with organized modern offensive and defensive weapons of malaria-warfare. The Panama, the Singapore and the Burma Campaign are well-known examples.

It is a fact that, despite intensive and extensive research, no drug or vaccine has yet been discovered which can cure malaria with certainty. It is hoped that more effective anti-malaria drugs may be found in the not too distant future, and that further researches may throw more light on the immunity factor in malaria. It is doubtful if it will ever be possible to get rid of malaria by curative measures. There is no doubt that malaria is a preventable disease, and already we possess enough knowledge to stamp it out of the country by organising control measures on proper lines. One of the greatest advances in preventive medicine one can wish for is to awaken the health conscience of the people, to enable them to take full share in the economic and industrial development of the country.

I have attempted in the following pages to give a brief account of the malaria problem in India. They were originally a few notes which I made while working in the field or laboratory, or for giving talks on malaria to officers and other ranks (medical and non-medical), or when reading reports of various malaria workers. The notes were later re-written in the form of an essay. They have now been revised and brought upto-date. These notes were not meant for publication but a number of friends who saw the manuscript urged that they should be published. This book is by no means a treatise on malaria nor does it claim to cover the extensive subject of malaria control. It is only a brief introduction to the malaria problem in India.

I am grateful to all those whose observations have been included in this book. Most of them have been cited in the references of the particular chapters. As some of the observations have been made from the notes kept by me it has not been possible to give the reference in each case. Lt. Col. Jaswant Singh, Director, Malaria Institute of India has given invaluable help in revising and rearranging the text.

I am indebted to Dr. K. Biswas, Major General Sir Gordon Covell, Dr. A.S. Erulker, Dr. P.M. Mehta, Dr. Jivraj Mehta, Dr. Baini Parsad, Dr. G. Ramsay and Sir Malcolm Watson for their help and advice. Acknowledgement is due to the Public Health Commissioner with the Government of India, Directors of Malaria Institute of India, the Imperial Agriculture Institute and School of Tropical Medicine, Calcutta, Directors of Public Health of Bihar, Bombay C. P., Madras, Punjab (pre-partition), NWFP, and Sind, and the Principal, Jaminibhushan Ashtanga Ayurveda Vidyalaya, Calcutta for providing valuable information : and to the Government of India Department of Health (now Ministry of Health) for the permission to reproduce parts of the Health Survey and Development Committee Report. My gratitude is also due to the University of Bombay and the Director, Medical Services Army in India, for the kind permission to publish this book and to Dr. Bisheshwar Prasad and Shrimati Saraswati Raina for reading the proofs.

B. L. R.

Simla,
January, 1951

CONTENTS

ILLUSTRATIONS

Sir Ronald Ross (1857-1932) *Frontispiece* courtesy National Institute of History of Medicine.

---

*From "Some Emergency Anti-malaria Measures" by Sir Malcolm Watson Courtesy Ross Institute of Tropical Hygiene London.

INTRODUCTION*

This brochure by Dr. Raina, which is an elaboration of the thesis he submitted to the University of Bombay and for which he was awarded the Dosabhai Cama prize by the Syndicate of the University is, as the title indicates, an "Introduction to the Malaria Problem in India". The author deals with the problem in various aspects. He explains it by saying that the heavy toll taken by, the disease whether of the civil population or of the Army is such as to make it imperative for the authorities to be less apathetic and the people less ignorant about it. The author has by facts and figures shown how greatly malaria contributes, both directly and indirectly to the high mortality as well as morbidity in this country. He has also shown that more soldiers have died of malaria than by enemy action and yet the author points out that more is done to combat disease like plague, cholera, etc. than to combat malaria. This neglect on the part of authority as well as of the people is due, as stated by the author, to the fact the havoc caused by malaria is not so glaringly perceptible as that caused by, say, plague or cholera. He is, therefore, right in bringing the fact to the public notice that apart from the high mortality due to malaria, it is a disease which, along with hookworm so widely distributed in rural areas, saps the vitality of the nation and is therefore a greater enemy of the people and must not be neglected any longer.

The author gives a brief but interesting history of the efforts made to find out the causes of malaria and also the various methods of combating it. He finally says, "The solution of the malaria problem in India requires serious consideration of

*First Edition.

five principal factors, *viz*. (1) education, (2) organization, (3) medical protection, (4) legislation, and (5) funds."

No one will dispute the fact that health education should form part of general education of the child. The non-recognition of this fact has made us pay heavily in men and money. The author, therefore, has done well to emphasise the fact.

There is also much to say in favour of the author's suggestion to include at least one question on the public health aspect of malaria in the University examination paper set in the subject of "Hygiene & Public Health" to make medical students and medical practitioners take a greater interest in malariology than they do at present.

The author's suggestion about setting up a central organisation in each Province as also the Central Board of Control for the whole country, to combat the disease is worth consideration. He is right when he says that the task of tackling the problem should not be left to local bodies who have neither the means nor the staff to undertake the work. The Governments, Central as well as Provincial, as also the Indian States should between them take up the responsibility of the preventive side of medicine and leave the curative side to the local bodies.

The author gives practical suggestions with regard to the measures to be adopted for the prevention of disease, suggestions both for the authorities concerned as well as the public. His is a useful treatise written in an easy style which I feel sure will be helpful to those concerned with the health of the nation.

Jivraj N. Mehta

Bombay
December, 1945

1

History

Malaria fever is not a new phenomenon in the medical history of India. Some of the earliest references to this fever occur in the *Atharva Veda* believed to have been composed about 1500 B.C. It was classified even in *Atharva Veda* according to the periodicity of attack of fever, *i.e.*, quotidian (*sadandim*), tertian (*tritiyakam*) and quartan (*vitrtiyam*). It was also classified according to the season in which the fever made its appearance, *viz.*, winter (*sitam*), summer (*graismam*) and rainy season (*varsikam*). It was common especially where there was excessive rain (*mahavrsah*) or too much grass (*mujavanta*). It also leads to the assumption that such fevers were common in *Gandhara* (Peshawar District and Hoti Mardan). *Anga* (country about Bhagalpur) and *Magadha* (Bihar State).

trtiyakam vitrtiyam sadandimuta saradam
takmanam sitam ruram graismam nasaya varsikam".

(A.V. V. 22.13)

"*oko asya mujavanta oko asya mahavrsah*
yavajjatastakmamstavanasi bahlikesu nyocarah".

(A.V. V. 22.5)

From the numerous references to it and analysis of its characteristics it would appear that malaria was the commonest type of fever. Its association with mosquito may be surmised by the descriptions which give nearly all the characteristics and habits of mosquitoes, especially needle like proboscis (*kusula*), bloody mouth (*lohitasyan*) and the habit of visiting the dwellings after sunset (*salah parinrtyanti sayam*). There is also reference to the use of odourous or fumigating medications used to destroy them.

In *ka* 5 *sukta* 22, reference is made to *takman*. Caraka and Susruta use the word *Jvara* for fever in general. It continues to be the group name of all diseases with fever as the main and dominating sign. These authors of the Ayurvedic period classify fever into five types instead of four of *Atharva Veda*, *viz.*, continuous (*Samtatah*), remittent (*Satatah*), quotidian (*Anyedyuskah*), tertian (*Trtiyakah*) and quartan (*Caturthakah*).

"ye salah prinartyanti sayam gardabhanadinah
kusula ye ca kuksilah kakubhah karubhah srimah
tanosadhe tvam gandhena visucinan vinasaya".

(A.V. VIII. 6.10)

"ye kukundhah kukurabhah krittirdursani bibhrati
kliba iva pranrtyanto vane ye kurvate ghosam tanito nasayamasi".

(A.V. VIII. 6.11)

"ye suryam na titiksanta atapantamamum divah
arayan bastivasino durgandhimllohitasyan makkan nasayamasi".

(A.V. VIII. 6.12)

"ye suryat parisarpanti snuseva svasuradadhim
bajasca tesam pingasca hrdaye'dhini vidhyatam".

(A.V. VIII. 6.24)

"Punah pancavidho drsto dosakalabalabalat
samtatah satato'nyedyustrtiyakacaturthakauh".

(Ca. Ci. 3.34)

"Anyedyuskah pratidinam dinam hitva trtiyakah
Dinadvayam yo visramya pratyeti sa caturthakah".

(Ca. Ci. 3.67)

"Saptaham va dasaham va dvadasahamathapi va
Santatya yo'visargi syat santatah sa nigadyate
Ahoratre satatako dvau kalavanuvartate
Anyedyuskastvahoratradekakalam pravartate
Trtiyakastrtiye' hni caturthe' hni caturthakah".

(Su. U. 39.69.70.71)

The similes given by these two authors to explain the advent and periodicity of this kind of fever are very significant. Caraka, for instance, compares the phenomena to the seed sown in the ground which takes one day to grow in case of quotidian, two days in case of tertian and three days in case of quartan; when they grow up they invade the whole body and not being counteracted by anti-bodies (*pratyanika*) they cause the fever. When the force of these invading elements is exhausted, they return to their original habitat and again begin to grow up. Susruta compares the advent of fever to the tide and ebb of the ocean. Caraka's account of the life history of malarial parasite is of special interest. Both the authors also state that this kind of fever is common in low land or land at the foot of the mountain. Besides these indirect references to malaria, we find in the *Susruta Samhita* a direct reference to five species of mosquitoes, *viz.*, sea-born, globular in shape, the huge type, black in colour and the mountainous. The bite of the mountainous species (*Parvatiya*) is stated to bear the same characteristics as that of deadly insects (*Pranahara Kita Damsana*) Later references to malaria mosquitoes or malarial fever in *Vagbhata*, *Madhava* and *Bhavamisra*, are simply repetitions of the statements made by these two authors. Presumably the use of mosquito-nets (*masakahari*) was also prevalent in India as would be evident from Marco Polo's account as early as the 13th A.D.

"Adhisete yatha bhumim bijam kale ca rahati
Adhisete tatha dhatum dosah kale ca kupyati
Sa vrdhim balakalam ca prapya dosastrtiyakam
Caturthakam ca kurute partyanikabalaksyat
Krtva veg am gatabalah sve sve sthane vyavasthitah
Punarvivrdhah sve kale jvarayanti naram malah".

(Ca. Ci. 3.68.69.70)

"*Yatha vegagame velam chadayitva mahodadheh*
Vegahanau tadevambhastatraivantarnitiyate
Dosavegodaye tadvadudiryete jvaro'sya vai
Vegahanau prasamyeta yatha mbhah' sagare tatha".

(Su. U. 39.73-74)

"*Masakah—samudrah, parimandalo, hastimaskah, krsnah, parvatiya iti panca; tairdastasya tivra kandur damsasothasca, parvatiyastu kitaih pranaharaistulyalaksanah.*"

(Su. Ka. 8.36)

It will be obvious, therefore, that malaria as a disease and its association with the mosquito was known as early as the Vedic period in ancient India. The word for mosquito in the *Atharva Veda* is *makka* which is the same as '*masaka*' in classical Sanskrit. The derivatives of the word mosquito in different Indo-European languages point out that an insect of this kind can be traced back to great antiquity*.

Fevers recurring periodically and cases with enlarged spleens were referred to by Hippocrates. Empedocles is reported to have freed Selinus from fever in 550 B.C. by draining the marshes. Egyptian, Greek, and Roman writers associated malaria with marshes and bad air. Varro, and Columella, about 116 B.C., refer to 'minute animals' and

Latin :—musca=a fly

Sanskriti :—Masaka=a mosquito from the root 'mas'=to hum

All these derivatives point to a common origin and this must be a word in the Indo-European language when the Aryan families had not migrated, one to Greece and the other to India, *i.e.*, before the splitting up of Indo-European language into Sanskrit, Greek, Latin, etc.

The words "paludal fever", "paludous", "paludism, meaning malarial fever, malarial living and malarial disease respectively, are derived from Latin *palus-udis* meaning marsh (*paludosus*: marshy). Sanskrit and Latin speaking scholars shared the view that malaria was associated with marshy regions.

'noxious streams' in marshes. Cicero wrote about a temple of fever Goddess in Palatine. Godfry of Viterbo commented on Roman fever: "*Those from whom Rome was unable to defend herself dispersed by the air. At whose breath the German youth fell*".

It was popularly believed that the cinchona bark for the treatment of malaria was brought to Europe by Countess of of Cinchon from Peru in 1640. A story often told was that Ana de Osoria, the first wife, of Francisca Henriquez de Ribera, the second wife, of Don Louis Geronimo Fernandez de Carera, the fourth Count of Cinchon, the Viceroy of Peru, was cured of fever about 1638 with powdered bark of quina-quina sent by a friend through her physician, Don Jaun de Vega, and later she took the bark to Europe. The official diary of the Count, however, discredits the popular story, as it reveals that the Countess, except for cough, never suffered from fever, nor ever took the bark to Europe, as she died in Columbia and never reached her home.

Haggis reported that later in the 16th and 17th centuries, Peruvian bark, quina-quina, was exported to Spain and Italy, which was later adulterated with another bark, cinchona. Heyden refers to the use of cinchona as early as 1643. The bark seemed to have been sent from Spain to Italy and England about 1655. Charles Marie de la Condamine, an astronomer, described the Peruvian tree, and in 1742 Carl von Linne, a Swedish botanist, gave the name cinchona to quina-quina tree. In 1820 the alkaloids, quinine and cinchonine, were isolated by two French pharmacists Pelletier and Caventou. In 1852 Justus Charles Hasskarl, a Dutch botanist, proceeded on an expedition to Bolivia and Peru, and two years later successfully started cinchona cultivation in Java. Clements R. Markham, a geographer, in 1860 took out a similar party, and later was responsible for starting cinchona plantation in the Nilgiri Hills near Ootacamund in Madras State. In 1865 a faithful servant of Charles Ledger collected for his master selected seeds of cinchona. Ledger sold them to planters in Madras and the Dutch. The Dutch developed the cinchona plantation, becoming the chief cinchona exporters, producing 20,000,000 pounds a year.

It seems that the treatment of malaria in India with cinchona was started in Calcutta about the year 1657. Dr. James Lind is reported to have treated with cinchona over 400 cases with very good results in 1765.

In 1804, Dr. James Johnson arrived in Calcutta and unfortunately could not cure his first patient with cinchona. His second case improved after bleeding. Johnson on his return to London wrote a book on tropical diseases, in which he strongly recommended his treatment based on a single case. Cinchona was given up and the treatment of bleeding and purging took its place. A typical course of treatment then was as follows :

1st day	bled	35 ounces	applied 20 leeches
2nd day	,,	20 ,,	,, 12 ,,
3rd day	,,	24 ,,	,, 6 ,,
4th day	,,	24 ,,	
5th day		½ gr. quinine repeated after one hour.	

The unfortunate patient was also given 55 grains of calomel, 46 grains of blue pill daily purges of colocynth, hyoscyamus, compound powder of jalap, camboge, senna and salts.

In 1893, Edward Hare arrived in India and observed that with the standard treatment of his days "patients all died, no remission took place, there were head symptoms, and he dared not give quinine, in fact it was utterly forbidden by all authorities that it never occurred to him to give it. Luckily soon after it occurred to him to give quinine and he dared to give it and successfully treated 700 cases of fever with a mortality of less than ½ per cent". Quinine soon came to the forefront again. It was used in various doses (20 gr., 45 gr., or 60 gr. daily) given for varying periods (26 days, 30 days, 18 days, 21 days and indefinitely) continuous or intermittent. Quinine appears to have been first used in India in or about 1826 and it was only by 1840 that its use was generally accepted. (Joglekar, 1940).

In 1847, Heinrich Meckel noticed grains of pigments in the blood vessels of the brain of patients suffering from malaria. In 1848 Virchow saw intracellular pigments. In 1875 Kelsch noted these pigmented bodies in the blood of patients suffering from malaria. On the 6th November 1880, Charles Louis Alphonse Laveran, a French Army, surgeon, described the malaria parasite at Constantine in Algeria. Italians considered them as degenerated red cells. They considered that *Bacillus malariae* isolated from water and soil by Klebs and Crudeli in 1879 was the causative organism. By 1885, Laveran's theory was accepted. In 1884 Gerhardt had produced an attack of malaria by injecting blood of malaria patient. Golgi and his collaborators, Marchiafava and Celle, in Italy reported different species of malaria parasites. Romanowsky's chromatin staining method since 1891 further facilitated observations and research. Koch distinctly showed three species of malaria.

It remained for Major Ronald Ross of the Indian Medical Service and Grassi and his colleagues to explode once and for all, the theory of malaria based on bad air and decomposing vegetation.* Ross when on short leave to Sigur Ghat in 1896, while investigating cases of malaria, found that 80% of the labourers had enlarged spleens. He had a severe attack of malaria himself before he returned to his duties in the army. On the constant persuasion of Sir Patrick Manson, (who, it may be stated, formulated the hypothesis of mosquito transmission theory in 1894 and stimulated the interest of Ross in the theory and showed him the malaria parasite for the first time in London Hospital) Ross continued his investigations. On the 20th

*Many consider, Grassi, as the greater pioneer. Comparison of great scientists is not always easy. Such quarrel "between the two was not worthy of scientists". Both Grassi and Ross were, no doubt, great pioneers. There are, however, reasons to feel that Grassi should recieve greater attention than is generally given to him.

August 1897, in Secunderabad, he made his epoch making discovery (demonstrating the malaria parasite in a mosquito that had fed on blood with malaria parasite) and completed on the 9th July 1898, the life cycle of the malaria parasite of avian malaria (*Plasmodium praecox*) in mosquitoes. Grassi, Bignami and Bastianelli worked out the complete development for human malaria in *Anopheles maculipennis* and transmitted the disease to man by the bite of the infected mosquito. Two years after, Sambon, Low and Terzi lived in a mosquito-proof house in Ostia, an intensely malarious locality in Roman Campagna, and remained free from malaria. Mosquitoes fed on malaria patients were sent from Rome to London and were made to bite other patients. Dr. P. Manson and Mr. George Warren volunteered and both of them developed severe attacks of malaria, leaving no doubt that malaria is caused by a parasite harboured in the blood of human beings and is caried from man to man by the female mosquito of a certain species. Full advantage of these discoveries was not taken for long despite the heavy toll taken by malaria.

In India, out of the total deaths in 1931, 60% were due to fever (⅓ at least being due to malaria) and only 5% were due to the much dreaded group of diseases like plague and cholera. Statistics covering the period 1932 to 1941 reveal that the malaria death rate approximates 37% of the total number of deaths in India.*

The incidence of malaria is of a still greater importance in war, as it often incapacitates more troops than battle casualties. Many military, operations have been brought to a standstill by malaria. Covell (1943) observed that "the very nature of an army's normal activities is such that almost every action it performs in a malarious country, is calculated to promote the spread of the disease, *viz.*, the constant movements of troops by night and day, the employment of large numbers of men on

*Positive cases of malaria in India in 1987 (provisional) reported were 1,663,284, with 185 deaths.

Source : National Malaria Eradication Programme, Delhi.

night duties, the difficulties of enforcing measures of personal protection, the aggregation of large bodies of labourers, the consequent introduction of new strains of malaria among the troops, the camping of troops in close proximity to malarious villages for strategic reasons, the dispersion of troops over large areas instead of concentrating them in easily protected camps, difficulties of transport, shortage of anti-malaria equipment and drugs, and the impossibility of ensuring that drugs are actually taken in the dosage and manner prescribed".

During the Walcheren expedition of 1809, out of 40,000, 4000 died from fever as against 668 killed in action. During the Rangoon expedition of 1804-05, there were only 35 deaths from wounds, but 450 out of every 1000 men engaged died of malaria. In the Burma expedition of 1824, the enterprise in Arakan had to be abandoned owing to fever "for everyone who was not dead was in hospital (75% of the whole force in action)". In 1916-18, malaria came into its own. In Macedonia, over 170,000 British troops were admitted to hospital (January to May 1916, 150 cases, June to December 1916, 30,000 cases, 1917, 70,000 cases, 1918, over 60,000 cases ; 25,000 resistant cases repatriated and two million days were lost). In East Africa, there were 107,702 admissions, giving the highest rate per thousand. Napoleon in 1809 is reported to have written to one of his ministers : "We rejoice to see that the English themselves are in the morasses of Zeeland ; only, keep them in check, and the bad air and fevers peculiar to the country will soon destroy them". In 1942, in Assam and Arakan (before anti-malaria measures were brought into full force) history once again repeated itself. In April 1942, a large railway project was rendered in—effective as 90% of the labourers were down with malaria. In the same year, a quarter of the force in the Assam front became casualties from a small winged enemy—*Anopheles minimus*. In 1943, ratio of casualties from wounds to sickness was 1 : 121. The total casualty rate per 1000 strength of India other ranks was 1128.9, *i.e.*, statistically evey soldier was more than once in hospital. Half the sick suffering from all diseases were suffering from malaria. In three months,

October to December 1942, 18,000 cases, mostly malaria, were evacuted by the Eastern Army. Field Marshal Lord Wavell instructed the G.O.Cs-in-C that "In theatres where future operations are likely to take place we may well find that disease and especially malaria is a more dangerous factor than enemy resistance. We have already had experience of the effects of a bad malarial season in Assam. We must prepare to meet malaria by training as strict and as earnest as against enemy troops. We must be as practised in the use of our weapons against it.........as we are with the rifle, we must study the habits of the mosquitoes as we do the tactics of the Japanese. We must know methods of anti-mosquito work as well as how to construct trenches to hold a position".

Soon after malaria control measures were taken, the malaria rate rapidly dropped. In 1945, malaria incidence was reduced to one-tenth of what it was in 1943. Over the whole Allied Land Forces South East Asia, the malaria sick rate dropped from 3.65 per 1000 to 0.20 per 1000. It can be confidently said that successful war against malaria was the major factor in the success of the Allies against the Japanese.

Effects of malaria in peace time are not so dramatic as of diseases like plague or cholera. Malaria imperceptibly, saps the vitality, diminishes normal expectation of life of those that survive, dislocates labour and industry, and retards the economic and social progress of the country as a whole. It has been responsible for accelerating the physical and intellectual degeneration of the people in tropics for centuries.

The live birth rate begins to fall after the malaria season sets in, and the reduction is most pronounced about a month after the epidemic is at its height. Watson (1924) pointed out that "when women get into a malarious locality, they rarely become pregnant and when pregnant soon abort". Brahmachari (1923) observed in a severe malaria epidemic that "apart from a rise in malaria mortality of 400, the recorded non-malaria death rate rises 2½ times". Malaria affects children and particularly those who are still in their teens, destroys their blood cells and renders them anaemic and stunted both physically and mentally. There can be no gainsaying that the malaria is one of the greatest problems which faces India.

It not only has a baneful influence on the growth of the population, but by lowering their vitality renders them more liable to contract other infections. It has been estimated that at least two million persons die in India every year due to the direct and indirect effects of malaria, and at least 125 to 175 million suffer from it, resulting in great loss of life, widespread misery, and in money 'unbelievable millions of pound sterling' annually (Sinton 1939).*

Malaria takes its toll in some places all the year round and in others seasonally and periodically. The Northern and Western parts of the Indo-Pakistan sub-continent show marked seasonal incidence. Christophers reported that during the 1908 epidemic "many villages and even whole Thanas showed high mortality during October and November—in some instances as high as 300, 400 and even 500 per mille". During years of abnormal epidemics total numbers of deaths may increase by ¼ to ½ million. The relatively recent, widespread epidemic occurred in 1942 and swept over a large area causing a very high morbidity and mortality.

Statistics to show the specific mortality rate directly due to malaria for all parts of India are not available. The following table may throw light on the incidence of malaria, as a fair proportion of fevers will be directly or indirectly due to malaria.

*This reflects the picture in 1939. In 1987 the incidence of malaria in India was less than 2 million and number of deaths due to malaria was 185.

Statement Showing Population, Density Per Square Mile, Birth Rate, Death Rate, Infantile Mortality Rate, Vital Index and Deaths from Fevers in British India Excluding Burma and the States During the Years 1928-1947*

Year	Density per sq. mile (Regn. areas only)	Birth rate per mille	Death rate per mille	Infantile mortality rate per 1000 live births	Vital index	Deaths from Fevers
1928	326	34.9	24.1	171.8	145	3352144
1929	330	33.2	42.2	176.8	137	3534357
1930	333	33.2	24.8	180.0	134	3703716
1931	328	34.6	25.1	178.0	138	3880799
1932	334	33.8	21.7	168.1	156	3380248
1933	339	35.5	22.3	169.7	159	3444483
1934	345	33.5	24.8	185.4	135	3[illegible]62910
1935	349	34.5	23.5	162.8	147	3666328
1936	360	34.9	22.3	161.0	157	3488521
1937	366	33.8	22.0	161.7	154	3569590
1938	370	33.3	23.7	167.1	141	3883627
1939	375	32.7	21.6	155 6	152	3613376
1940	380	32.0	21.1	159.8	152	3622072
1941	385	32.1	21.8	158.0	147	3697541
1942	388	29.5	21.4	162.6	138	3794245
1943	390	26.1	23.9	164.7	109	4138751
1944	391	25.8	24.5	169.3	105	4352143
1945	393	28.0	22.1	150.9	127	3832479
1946	397	28.9	18.7	136.4	154	2821598
1947**	406	26.6	19.7	145.6	135	2587317

**The recent population figures for India are* Density of population including projected population of Assam : population (1981 census) 685 184,692. 216 per Km² ; Crude Birth Rate 1986 (provisional) : 32.4 (rural 34.1 and urban 27.0) ; Crude Death Rate 1986 (provisional) : 11.1 (rural 12.1 and urban 7.6) ; Infant Mortality 1986 : 96 (rural 105 and urban 62).

Source : Verma, V.S. *Census of India, A Handbook of Population Statistics.* First Users Conference for 1991 Census. Office of the Registrar General & Census Commissioner India, New Delhi, 1988.

**Indian Union Provinces as after partition only.

Statistics are often impressive, especially vital statistics. But this science of numbers, applied to the life history of the people of India, has its limitations. 400 million people inhabiting the Indian sub-continent,* mostly live in its 700,000 villages, where large numbers of deaths, births and diseases are inaccurately recorded and reported. Malaria is mostly, reported on clinical grounds in urban dispensaries. The main bulk of the information in rural areas is collected by a petty village official (*Chowkidar*), who is not likely to report cases with any degree of scientific accuracy. It is, however, noticeable that the problem of malaria varies from place to place, and with notable exceptions in isolated controlled areas, has not appreciably lessened. Sinton's observations made years ago, "the problem of existence in very many parts of India is the problem of malaria" is true even today.**

*Population of India estimate for mid 1990 : about 853.4 million. *Source* : 1990 population data sheet Population Reference Bureau Inc., Washington.

**The malaria situation improved after National Malaria Control Programme was launched in April 1953. In 1947, the incidence of malaria in India after Independence, was estimated as about 75 million, with about 0.8 million deaths. The results of National Malaria Control Programme, later developed as National Malaria Eradication Programme in 1958 were very encouraging upto 1965. The incidence gradually increased for various reasons during 1966-76. A decline in malaria cases is reported since 1981.

Positive Malaria Cases

Year	Cases	Deaths
1961	49,151	nil
1966	148,015	nil
1971	1,322,398	nil
1976	6,467,215	59
1981	2,701,141	170
1986	1,792,167	323
1987 (provisional)	1,663,284	185

Health Information India, p. 154, CBHI Directorate General Health Service, New Delhi, 1988. *Source* : NMEP Delhi.

REFERENCES

Brahmachari, B.B., (1923) *Verification of vital statistics in certain typical areas of Murshidabad, Calcutta.*

Christophers, S. R., (1911) *Sc., Mem. Off. Med. and Sanit. Depts.,* Government of India (New series), No. 46.

Covell, G., (1941) *Health Bulletin 5, Malaria Bureau No. I.* Manager Publications, Delhi.

Covell., G., (1943) *J. Mal. Inst. Ind.* 5, 129.

Joglekar, G. V., (1940) *I. M. J*, Vol. 34, No. 11, Vol. 35. Nos. 1 & 2.

Sinton, J. A., (1939) *Health Bulletin No. 26, Malaria Bureau No. 13,* Manager Publication, Delhi.

Watson, M., (1924) *Report on the Health of Tea Gardens situated in Upper Assam with special reference to malaria.*

2

The Parasite

There are four species of malaria parasites of the genus *Plasmodium—Plasmodium vivax* (Grassi and Feletti 1890) causing benign tertian malaria, *P. malariae* (Laveran 1880-81) quartan malaria, and *P. falciparum* (Welch 1897) malignant tertian malaria. There is a fourth plasmodium called *P. ovale* (Stephens, 1922).* *P. ovale* is rare and almost limited to Africa and causes mild tertian fever. Each of these has a sexual cycle in the female anopheline mosquito, the exo-erythrocytic cycle in the liver of human beings and erythrocytic cycle in the blood stream. The different types of plasmodia differ in morphology, but their history is essentially the same. The parasite in man undergoes a series of changes. It is seen like a pale disc on or within a red blood cell, with black or reddish black particles scattered in the cytoplasm. Particles collect in the centre, round which the cytoplasm arranges itself into segments. Finally, the red blood cells break down, liberating the segments, callen merozoites. These merozoites adhere to other red cells, enter them and grow at the expense of the haemoglobin, and repeat the same cycle. After several generations of merozoites, a few develop into sexual forms

***P. tenue* (Stephens, 1914) is of a doubtful species. Man has also been experimentally infected with *P. knowlesi*, a parasite of monkeys.

(male or macro and female or micro gametocytes). The sexual forms cannot develop any further in the human body. When taken by a specific mosquito, macro and microgametocytes join and form a zygote. The zygote bores its way through the epithelium of the stomach of the mosquito, encysts between the epithelium and the limiting membrane and becomes an oocyst in which numerous slender motile spindle shaped bodies about 12-15μ called the sporozoites are formed. The oocyst ruptures when liberating the sporozoites into the caelomic cavity. These sporozoites are motile and get collected in the salivary glands of the mosquito and are injected with the salivary secretion into the human body when the mosquito next feeds. The history of human malaria parasite after being injected into man by the mosquito till it appears in the circulating red blood cells remained a mystery till recently. Shortt *et. al.* (1948a) reported the pre-erythrocytic forms of *P. cynomolgi* (a malaria parasite of the monkeys) in liver on the sixth and seventh days of incubation period. It was assumed that the life of *P. vivax* in man would resemble that of *P. cynomolgi* as seen in the liver of *Macaca mulata*. The above presumption was finally proved at Horton hospital, Epsom, where a large number of *A. maculipennis atroparvus* infected with *P. vivax* were fed upon a patient and isolated salivary glands of the infected mosquitoes were inoculated intravenously into the same patient. The biopsy was performed several days after. The material examined showed plasmodial masses studded with chromatin particles very similar in appearance to those previously, seen in the case of infection of the monkey with *P. cynomolgi*. The forms seen measured up to 42 μ in diameter and showed in some instances the vacuoles noted in the case of *P. cynomolgi*. (Shortt *et. al.*, 148b).

Thus, the asexual and sexual forms of the malaria parasite develop in man and mosquito respectively. The infected red cells in man rupture and release the merozoites to infect fresh cells. This coincides with the rise of temperature and shivering. The attack of fever may occur in one type (quartan) every 72 hours or every 4th day: in the other two types (benign and malignant tertian) every 48 hours or every third day, and in still other types daily or at irregular intervals (mixed infection). A person gets fever after not less than 10 to 14 days of the bite of the mosquito. About 10 days after the attack of fever, the sexual forms mature in man. If the mosquito of the carrier species feeds on an infected man having these sexual forms, it takes the parasite about two weeks to develop into the sporozoite provided climatic conditions are suitable for maturation of the malaria parasite in the mosquito and the blood feed has been taken from a person carrying the sexual forms which are fully mature.

The infected cell becomes enlarged in size in *P. vivax* infection. The infected erythrocytes of *P. falciparum* clump together and adhere to the walls of the capillaries, leading to serious complications associated with malignant subtertian infection. Another notable feature of *P. falciparum* infection is that the cells may be infected with three or more sets of parasites concurrently each causing a continuous paroxysm of fever.

The incubation period differs in the different species, about a week to 12 days in malignant tertian, about two weeks in benign tertian and about three weeks in quartan infection.

Benign tertian infection is usually of a persistent type though it may have a low parasite count. Symptoms are usually mild, despite chill and high fever, and paroxysms last for about ten hours. *P. vivax*, like *P. falciparum*, can sometimes give rise to severe cerebral symptoms. (Dhayagude and Purandare, 1943). Joint pains, herpes labialis and gastro-intestinal symptoms, especially vomiting, are often noted. Malaria cases with symptoms of acute intestinal obstruction have been described. Relapses after as many as 10 to 20 years have been recorded. Rigors with fever are seen in both benign tertian and quartan. Nephritis has been occasionally found. Hyperpyrexia is seen especially with *P. falciparum* infection and is a dangerous symptom. Paroxysms of fever may last twenty to thirty hours and may show a double peak and no chill. Mild febrile attacks of long duration, anaemia, black water fever, together with pneumonic, cardiac, psychotic and algid types, are not uncommon in the tropics.

The parasites show regional distribution and seasonal preference. One species may be prevalent in one season and another at a different period, due to variations of temperature and humidity at different times. If meteorological conditions remain uniform, no change may be observed.

P. vivax, seems to predominate from March to July and *P. falciparum* from July to December, reaching maximum incidence in May and October, respectively.

In areas where only one species of parasite is predominant, infection with the predominant species is found, and in those areas where two or three parasites are found, a person can be infected with one or more of them. Different seasonal changes too may affect prevalence of mixed infection. Gametocytes also show variations. It is stated that relative output is lowest in *P. falciparum*; on the other hand, its increased rate of shizogony ensures that its absolute output of gametocytes is higher than in either of the other two species. Knowles *et. al.* suggest that the proportion of gametocytes may depend on long duration of infection, age of patient (basal metabolism), administration of drugs and the season of the year when examination is made. Mixed infections constitute about 3.7% of the general malaria of the world, and may be distributed as follows:—

P. vivax plus *P. malariae* 9.1%, *P. vivax* plus *P. falciparum* 79%, *P. malariae* plus *P. falciparum* 10.4%, *P. vivax* plus *P. malariae* plus *P. falciparum* 1.5%.

Knowles *et. al.* (1930) give the following distribution :

Provinces	P. vivax	P. malariae	P. falci-parum	Mixed	No. examined	No. positive
N.W.F.P.	... 37.8%	0.3%	61.9%	5.0	17,000	8814
Punjab	... 58.4%	1.0%	40.6%	...	2,707	2210
Delhi	... 54.4%	1.2%	44.4%	...	1,694	1139
Rajputana	... 90.0%	...	10.0%	...	...	...
U.P. including Nepal	... 70.0%	3.9%	26.1%	7.0	5,843	1830
C.P.	... 59.0%	11.8%	30.2%	...	2,209	995
Bombay including Goa	... 55.4%	5.9%	38.7%	5.6	16,275	7437
Mysore State	... 69.4%	2.0%	28.6%	...	1,900	559
Hyderabad Deccan	... 35.6%	9.7%	54.5%	...	...	174
Coorg	... 28.0%	24.0%	48.0%	...	...	416
Madras Presy.	57.8%	7.0%	35.2%	...	4,596	1699
Agency Tracts	41.0%	41.0%	18.0%	...	...	575
Bihar Orissa	... 49.4%	1.2%	49.2%	4.0	1,478	722
Bengal Presy.	41.4%	12.3%	46.3%	265	19,860	8520
Assam	... 36.3%	9 9%	53.9%	74	over 7,814	3068

This gives an over all distribution as follows as in 1930 :—

P. vivax	...	47.1%
P. malariae	...	6.9%
P. falsiparum	...	45.9%

The average gametocyte output of the three species (Calcutta findings) is, for *P. vivax* 21.2%, *P. malariae* 44.7%, *P. falciparum* 18.9%. Great variations are found, especially in the case of *P. falciparum* (Knowles *et. al.*). It may be added that the distribution of the various species is not clearly understood. Distribution of *P. malariae* in general seems to be limited by summer isotherm of 60°F., *P. falciparum* by 70°F., *P. malariae* appears to be a dying species; maximum output of *P. falciparum* occurs often towards the close of transmission period.*

Deaderick reported the following percentages of relapses:—

P. vivax	...	...	65%
P. malariae	...	...	55%
P. falciparum	...	...	45%

It will be seen that all plasmodia can cause further acute attacks of malaria. *P. vivax* relapses are extremely common and the relapse rate is probably higher than quoted above. The study of therapeutically induced malaria shows that benign tertian relapses occur first within three months of the primary attack and the second between the sixth and the ninth month of the first attack, and the malignant tertian relapses within three months of the first attack. It may be added that lower bodily resistance from disease or malnutrition, chill, overexertion and fatigue also tend to precipitate relapses.

REFERENCES

Dhayagude, R.G. and Purandare, N.M., (1943) *Arch, Pathology*, 36, 550-58.

Knowles, R., Senior White, R. and Das Gupta, B.M., (1930) *Ind. J. Med. Res. Mem.*, 18, 43-101, 298, 306.

Shortt, H. E Garnham, P. C. C. and Malamos, B., (1948a) *Brit. Med. J.*, Jan, 31, 192.

Shortt, H. E. Garnham, P. C. C., Covell, G. and Shute, P. G., (1948b) *Ibid.*, March 20, 547.

*In 1987, the distribution of *P. falciparum* was reported as about 37 per cent of all malaria cases.

3

The Mosquito

There are approximately 1700 species of mosquitoes in the world; but of these only about 180 are anophelines, and out of these about 17 only are important carriers of malaria. Forty three species and, variants of anopheline mosquitoes have been identified in India and Pakistan,* out of which about 7 are chief vectors of this disease and a few others are of lesser importance.

In their life cycle,** all mosquitoes pass through four stages of development. The fertilized eggs are laid by the adult female mosquito on water. Anopheline eggs are boat shaped and are laid singly and have distinctive markings. They develop into larvae which lie parallel to the surface of the water. They feed on aquatic vegetation, dead or living, and on animal life. The larvae moult four times in two days to several months and after their fourth moult develop into comma-shaped pupae. For a few hours to as much as a few days the pupae rest on

*India, Pakistan and Bangladesh.

**About 60 species of *Anopheles* have been incriminated in the world as carriers, but there may be others not yet reported. The *Anophelini* and *Culicini* eggs, larvae pupae and adults can be distinguished from the following characteristics:

(*Contd. on next page*)

the surface of water; the skin then splits and the adult mosquito emerges. The duration of the aquatic phase of development depends, among other factors, on the climatic conditions. It will be seen that about ten days in each case are required for the (*a*) development of eggs to mosquito, (*b*) development of parasite in the mosquito, and (*c*) incubation period of parasite in man.

The malaria carriers widely differ in their habits and distribution. The adult mosquitoes as well as the larvae of different species can be identified from one another on morphological characters. The distribution, breeding places and habits of some of them are briefly described below:

Important Malaria Carriers*

A. culicifacies Giles 1901; It is the chief malaria carrier

(*Contd. from previous page*)

	Anophelini	*Culicini*
Eggs	Boat shaped Dorsolateral floats transversely or radially arranged, Collect into clumps giving triangular and star shapes.	Micropilar spinous process at head end. Collect in drafts of hundreds of eggs.
Larvae	Aperture on 8th abdominal segment.	Long or short syphon tube on 8th abdominal segment.
	Float parallel to the surface of water.	Float head down with syphon tube on surface.
Pupae	Spiracles, short stumpy and funnel shaped.	Spiracles, longer, slender and trumpet shaped.
Adult mosquitoes	Long and club shaped palpi in male. Palpi as long as *Probocis* in female. When resting appear to stand on its head except a few species.	Long and tapering palpi in male. Palpi bud like shorter than *Probocis* In female *Probocis* bent at angle with body. Rest parallel to the surface.

*Of the numerous publications consulted Notes on the Distribution, Breeding Places. Adult Habits and Relation to Malaria of the Anopheline Mosquitoes of India and Far East (Covell, 1944) were of great help in prepating this account.

of the northern plains of Indo-Pakistan sub-continent,* but is of no practical importance in East** and West Bengal and Assam. It breeds in swamps (produced by floods), in irrigation channels, rain water pools, pools in pebble-bedded rivers, slow streams, rice and fallow fields, tanks and swimming pools. Chalam (1926) found it breeding in brackish waters. The adult mosquito is found in houses and cowsheds. It feeds on human and bovine blood indifferently (Covell and Jaswant Singh, 1943) and has an average flight range of ½ to 1 mile. Temperatures between 25°C. and 30°C. with 60% relative humidity are the most favourable conditions for its longevity and general activity.

A. fluviatilis James 1902: It is widely distributed throughout India and Pakistan*** and is the chief malaria carrier in the foot-hills of Southern India, the Kanara and Thana districts of Bombay State, Hazaribagh ranges, all places on or at the foot of Sabudris (part of Western Ghats) and in parts of Uttar Pradesh. It is rare in Assam, and generally speaking, is of little importance in North India and Pakistan. It breeds in clear water, seepages, streams with grassy margins, springs, edges of lakes, swamps, tanks and irrigation channels of terraced rice fields. It is mostly found above 1000 feet but not commonly above 5000 feet above sea level. Breeding places are usually within 1500 feet of habitations in Wynad. South India (Adisubramaniam and Vedmanikkam, 1943) but have been reported up to 2400 feet from human habitation in the Kangra Valley (Raina, 1944). Adults feed mostly on human beings in Wynad (South India) but mainly on cattle in the Uttar Pradesh. In North Kanara District, it is reported that this species takes its blood before midnight; feeding may commence within 1½ hours after dusk (Viswanathan and Rao, 1943). It has been reported to feed in the Satpuras at 2 A.M. (Senior White, 1941) whereas biting during the day has been reported in the Jeypore Hill tract (Perry 1914).

*Bangladesh, India and Pakistan.

**Bangladesh.

***Bangladesh, India and Pakistan.

A. minimus Theobald 1901 : This is the chief vector of Eastern Assam and Northern Bengal. This species has also been recorded from Bihar, Chhota Nagpur, Hyderabad, Konkan, Madras, Malabar, Mysore State, Orissa and the foot-hills of the Himalayas up to Uttar Pradesh. It breeds in grassy-edged, clear, cool and slow running streams, rivers, drains, exposed seepages, *kuchha* wells, irrigation chanels of the rice fields, occasionally in grassy edged pools, burrow-pits and tanks during the cold period of the year. It does not breed under dense shade or in highly polluted drains from factories. Shade itself plays no direct part in control. The absence of larvae is entirely due to secondary effects, due to shading, *viz.* grass not growing at the edges under dense shade. Muirhead Thomson (1940) observed that eggs are laid normally at night. Sixty-nine per cent of oviposition takes place during the first third of the night, twenty-two per cent in the middle third, and nine per cent in the last third. In the selection of a breeding place, illumination at night is a more useful expression of light factor than daylight or sunlight. The gravid female is strongly attracted by shade and will not oviposit in an unshaded position. Although *A. minimus* breeds in association with running water with grassy edges, where eggs are laid and where the larvae breed, the water is usually still. Ovipositing females avoid flowing water even when the velocity is as low as one foot in 20 seconds. Larvae are unable to resist a current velocity greater than 0.29 foot per second. The larvae are also strongly attracted to shade. This attraction is so great that the larvae will leave unshaded zones of still water in favour of shaded zones where the current may be sufficient to flush them downstream. The thermal death point of the larvae is 41°F. The maximum water temperature of typical *A. minimus* running water breeding places seldom exceeds 35°C. It is very sensitive to pollution by decomposing vegetation and this sensitivity may be one of the deciding factors for the gravid female to avoid oviposition in polluted water collections. The relation of ferruginous water to breeding places seems to depend on lack of food (algae) for the larvae, and not to any larvicidal action of colloidal iron. Silt by *itself* has no marked lethal action on *A. minimus larvae.* The controlling effect attributed to silt is due to increase in current velocity. *A. minimus* lays more eggs in the monsoon, but their expectation of life is greater at the end of the rainy season. In the hot damp monsoon, *A. minimus* takes two days to digest a blood meal and develop its ovaries ; ovipositing occurs in the second night after feeding. In cold weather this period is increased to 4-6 days. In the dry zones of the Dooars the most important breeding places during cold weather are perennial seepages and small streams. It feeds mostly on human beings. Dark houses are preferred as resting places and 90 per cent of feeding takes place after midnight. Natural infections are high during the months of March, June, August and September.

A. philippinensis Ludlow 1902 : This species is found in Assam, East* and West Bengal, Bihar, Bombay, Deccan, Chhota Nagpur, Konkan, Madras Coast, North Malabar, Mysore and Orissa. It is an important vector in the plains of Bengal where in clear, cool, stagnant water with aquatic vegetation (especially *Hydrilla verticillata, Ceratophyllum demersum, Utricularia* and *Najas*), nonfilamentous green algae, exposed to sunshine. Duck-weed, water hyacinth, blue-green algae (*Anabaena* and *Oscillatoria*), algae of family Cynophyceae, especially *Microcystis aeruginosa* are inhibitory to breeding of the larvae. Subsoil water seems to bear inverse relation to the density of the breeding ; the lower the subsoil water level the higher is the density of this species. In East* and West Bengal the adult mosquito is found mainly in human habitations (Krishnan, 1940 : Iyengar, 1944). In Assam, however, it is zoophilic and is normally found in cattle sheds (Ramsay, 1944). The usual resting places in the houses are on the wall within a few feet of the floor. They bite usually from 8 P.M. to 10 P.M. and 2 A.M. to 4 A.M.

A. stephensi Liston 1901 : This species is a vector in Western, North-western Peninsula, and Northern parts of Indo-Pakistan sub-continent, Bombay City, Bangalore, parts

*Bangladesh.

of Uttar Pradesh, Tanna Tracts of Chinwari District, Bhausi Tract of Amraoti District and Rupzar Tract of Balaghat. It breeds in wells, tins, roof gutters, tanks tubs, seepages, swamps, marshes and irrigation channels. It can breed in water contaminated with sewage (Roy, 1931). It has been reported breeding in salt pans during September and October in Bombay (Bana, 1943). Adults are strong fliers and may fly up to about 3 miles.

A. stephensi var *mysorensis* Sweet and Rao, 1937 : It is found in Poona, Sind, Vizagapatam, Mysore State and usually breeds in irrigation channels, margins of streams and wells. It is the chief rural carrier of malaria in Vizagapatam (Senior White, 1943).

A. sundaicus Rodenwaldt 1926 : It is found on the Arakan coast, in Sunderbans, in Hoogly Estuary, Coastal Belt of Orissa, Coastal Regions of Burma, lower Bengal, Madras State, in salt lakes of Calutta and Vizagapatam.* It breeds in brackish water, partially cleared mangrove swamps, artificial basins in which tidal water and fresh water mix and is often associated with algae (*Enteromorpha, Cladophora, Cyanophceae*), *Oscillatoria germinata, Lyngbya confervoides, Oedogoniumsp* and dead aquatic vegetation (*Potamogeton pectinatus, Halophila ovata* bound by alga *Lyngbya aestuarii*). They bite both in the day and night, feed on human beings and can fly for about a mile for their food.

CARRIERS OF LOCAL IMPORTANCE

A. annularis Van der Wulp 1884 : It is a carrier in parts of Bengal and Orissa Coastal Plain (Senior White and Rao, 1943). It has once been reported infected in nature, at Ferozepur (Adie, 1903). It breeds in still stagnant waters and pools, tanks, burrow-pits, and is often found associated with floating vegetation (*Hydrilla verticillata, Ceratophyllum demersum*) and algal growth (*Spirogyra*). Even slow movement of water is not favoured by its larvae. The adults are found in houses in maximum number during August or September and in cowsheds during October and November. During September-October

*also in Andaman and Nicobar Islands.

and the first half of November, the adults appear to live longer and feed on human beings in preference to cattle.

A. jeyporiensis var. *candidiensis* Koidzumi 1933 : This species is found in Assam, Bengal, Utter Pradesh and Malabar. Iyengar (1934) reported 4 gut infections out of 3833 dissected in Travancore. It has been reported infected in nature in extreme South East Bengal (Arakan). It breeds in slow running streams and rivers with grassy edges, also in lakes, swamps, seepages and ditches.

A. leucosphyrus Donitz 1901 : It is found in Assam, Bengal, Konkan, Madras, Malabar and Mysore State. It is reported to be a carrier in Digboi, Assam (Clark and Chaudhury, 1941). It usually breeds in partially shaded slow-running grassy edged streams. It feeds freely on human beings in Assam ; 75% out of 102 examined were found with human blood (Ramsay *et. al.*, 1936).

A. maculatus Theobald 1901 : This species is widely distributed in the submontane tracts in the North, South and East of Indo-Pakistan sub-continent, and along the foot of the Himalayas up to 8,000 feet. It breeds in streams, pools and river beds, in sunshine and feeds principally on cattle. It bites human beings between 9 P.M. and 2 A.M. after which it leaves the houses, rests outdoors under stream banks (Venhuis, 1941) and is of no real importance.

A. superpictus Grassi 1899 : It has been reported in Baluchistan, Waziristan and the N.W.F.P.* It has not been found east of the river Indus. Its favourite breeding places are seepages, rivers, streams, irrigation channels, reservoirs and springs It appears to have marked preference for running water exposed to sunlight, especially along the edges of streams and masses of spirogyra. The adult mosquito rests outdoors in caves, *karezes*.

A. varuna Iyengar 1924 : It is found in Assam, Bengal, Bihar, Bombay, Chhota Nagpur, Gujarat, Konkan, Madras

*Pakistan.

East Coast, Malabar, Mysore, Orissa and Uttar Pradesh. It has been found infected in nature in Travancore (Mathew, 1939), Hooghly Delta (Iyengar, 1928), Calcutta (Roy, 1939), Jeypore Singhbhum Hills, and appears to be of no importance elsewhere. It seems that there are two different biological races, one in eastern coast of India and the other in the hills of Central India and Bengal Delta. It breeds in terraced rice fields, irrigation channels, streams, seepages and roadside storm water drains. Adults are found in cowsheds and human habitations.*

Carriers of Little or no Importance

A. aconitus Donitz 1902 : This is found in Assam, Bengal, Bihar, Madhya Pradesh, Hyderabad, Konkan, Madras North Coast, Malabar, Orissa and Uttar Pradesh. Two specimens were reported infected (1 gut, 1 gut and gland) out of 24 dissected at Chandpur, Bengal (Das, 1943). One gut infection was reported from Jeypore Hills out of 107 dissected (Senior White, 1937), and one gut infection out of 1145 dissected from Lakhimpur, Goalpara District. It breeds in swamps, ponds, irrigation channels, rice fields, roadside drains and tanks with grassy margins. Adults are found in houses and cowsheds.

A. jeyporiensis James 1902 : This is found in Assam, Bengal, Bombay, Deccan, Central India, Madhya Pradesh, Uttar Pradesh, Chhota Nagpur, Gujarat, Hyderabad State, Konkan, Madras State, Malabar and Mysore State. Two gut infections, out of 674 dissected in Mysore State were found (Nursing, Rao and Sweet, 1934). Senior White (1937) reported four gut infections out of 318 dissected in Jeypore Hill Tract. Ramsay *et. al* (1936) recorded one gut infection out of 3115 dissected. It breeds in streams, irrigation channels, edges of ponds and lakes. Adults are mostly found in cattle sheds.

A. karwari James 1903 : This species is found in Assam, Bengal, Bihar, Bombay, Deccan, Chhota Nagpur, Konkan,

******A.b. balabacensis*** **in North-Eastern India forest areas has also been reported as a vector of local importance.**

Malabar, Mysore State and Orissa. One gut infection out of 125 specimens dissected in Assam (Strickland, 1929) and no infection in 15000 dissected (Ramsay *et. al.*, 1936) have been reported. It breeds in springs, pools, cool stream, swamps and seepages. Adults are found both in cattle sheds and human habitation, but mainly feed on cattle.

A. kochi Donitz 1901 : Ramsay. (1930) reported only, two gut infections out of 77 dissected in July at Cachar, Assam (total dissected in the year 2113). It breeds in small pools, irrigation channels, streams, containers and split bamboos. It feeds both on men on and animals.

A. pallidus Theobald 1901 : It has been reported infected in nature from Chanda, Madhya Pradesh (Kenrick, 1914), Krishnagar, Bengal (24 per cent gut infection, Sur and Sur, 1929) Birnagar, Bengal (Bose, 1931), Birbhum, Bengal (0.03% sporozoite rate, Timbres, 1935). Udaipur State (0.7 per cent gland infection, Roy and Biswas, 1942). Senior White and Adhikari, 1940 reported only four infected out of 3157 dissected in the East Satpura Ranges. It breeds in burrowpits, rice fields and tanks. Adults are mostly found in cattle sheds.

A. pulcherrimus Theobald 1902 : It breeds in swamps, pools and collections of stagnant water. Adults are frequent in both cattle sheds and human habitation. It is a strong flier.

A. ramsayi Covell 1927 : Only one gland infection was reported out of 217 dissected in Assam by Ramsay in 1930. No further infection has been reported (Ramsay, 1943). It is found in Assam, Bengal, Bihar, and Orissa and breeds in tanks, pools and swamps with vegetation, especially *Pistia stratiotes*. Adult mosquitoes rest in both cowsheds and human habitation.

A. splendidus Koidzumi 1920 : It has been reported infected in nature from Saharanpur (Robertson, 1910) and Karnal (Macdonald and Majid, 1931). It breeds in small pools seepages, tanks and streams with algae. Adults are found in cattle sheds and houses.

A. subpictus Grassi 1899 : It has been reported infected in nature at Pattukkottai, Madras State (1 gut and 1 gut and gland infection out of 13277 dissected Russell and Rao, 1940). Two gut infections were also found positive in Ennore out of 4728 dissected (Russell and Jacob, 19 9). It breeds in collections of water, burrow-pits, roof gutters, containers, sewage, polluted pools and even in brackish water. Adults mostly feed on cattle and are found both in houses and cattle sheds.

A. vagus Donitz 1902 : It is found in Assam, Bengal, Bihar, Bombay, Deccan, Madhya Pradesh, Chhota Nagpur, Gujarat, Hyderabad, Konkan, Madras East and West Coast, Malabar, Mysore State and Orissa. It has been reported infected in nature from Pattukkottai, S. India (one gland infection out of 6874 dissected, Russell and Rao *loc. cit.*) and from Assam (2 gland infections out of 10452 dissected, Strickland *et. al.*, 1933). It breeds in small pools, and is found in houses and cattle sheds, but feeds mostly on animals.

The following additional species of anophelines have been reported in India but natural infection in them have not yet been reported :

A. aitkeni, A. aitkeni var. *bengalensis, A. annandalei, A. annandalei* var. *interruptus, A. barbirostris, A. barbirostris* var. *anouni, A. barianensis, A. culiciformis, A. dthali, A. gigas, A. gigas*, var. *baileyi, A. gigas* var. *refutans, A. gigas* var. *simlensis, A. hyrcanus, A. insulaeflorum, A. jamesi, A. lindesayi* var. *nulgiricus, A. majidi, A. moghulensis, A. multicolor, A. pinjaurensis, A. sergenti, A. sintoni, A. tessellatus, A. theobaldi, A. turkkhudi* and *A. umbrosus.*

The following are known vectors in the neighbouring countries :

Burma : *A. minimus, A. jeyporiensis* var. *candidiensis, A. sundaicus, A. annularis.*

Malaya : *A. sundaicus, A. maculatus, A. umbrosus.*

Java :	*A. sundaicus, A. aconitus.*
Sumatra :	*A. sundaicus, A. aconitus, A. hyrcanus* var. *sinensis, A. leucosphyrus, A. umbrosus, A. kochi, A. subpictus, A. barbirostris.*
Indo-China and Eastern and Southern China	*A. minimus A. jeyporiensis* var. *candidiensis, A. hyrcanus* var. *sinensis, A. sundaicus, A. subpictus*, var. *indefinitus.*

REFERENCES

Adie, J.R., (1903) *Ind. Med. Gaz.*, 38, 246-249.

Adisubiramaniam, T.S. and Vedamamkkam, F.C., (1943) *J. Mal. Inst. Ind.*, 5, 113-116.

Bana, F.D., (1943) *Ibid.*, 123-124.

Bose, K., (1931) *Rec. Mal. Surv. Ind.* 2, 193-224.

Chalam, S.S., (1926) *Ind. Med. Gaz.*, 61, 375-376.

Clark, R.H.P. and Choudhury, M.A., (1941) *J. Mal. Inst. Ind.* 4, 103-107.

Covell, G. and Jaswant Singh, (1943) *Ibid.*, 5, 87-106.

Covell, G., (1944) *Ibid.*, 5, 399-434.

Das, B. K., (1943) *Ind. Med. Gaz.*, 78, 327-330.

Iyengar, M.O.T., (1928) *Report on the malaria survey of the environs Calcutta*, Government Press, Calcutta.

Idem., (1934) *Rec. Mal. Surv. Ind.*, 4, 61-63.

Idem., (1944) *J. Mal. Inst. Ind.*, 5, 435-448.

Kenrick, W. H., (1914) *Report upon malaria in the Central Provinces* 1912-13, Government Press, Nagpur.

Krishnan, K. V., (1940) *Report of the Prof. of entomology and rural hygiene*. Rept. All India Inst. Hyg. Publ. Health, 1939, 32-36.

Macdonald, G. and Majid, A., (1931) *Rec. Mal. Surv. Ind.*, 2, 423-480.

Matthew, M. I., (1939) *J. Mal. Inst. Ind.* 2, 101-104.

Muirhead Thomson, R. C., (1940) *Ibid.*, 3, 293, 294, 321, 322, 347, 348 and 4, 100-101, 244, 254.

Nursing, D., Rao, B.A. and Sweet, W.C., (1934) *Rec. Mal. Surv. Ind.* 4, 243-251.

Perry, E.L., (1914) *Ind. J. Med. Res.* 2, 456-491.

Raina, B. L., (1944) *Malaria Survey Yol. Kangra Valley*—(Not published).

Ramsay, G. C., (1930) *Ind. J. Med Res.* 18, 533-552.

Idem., (1941) *Report of the Committee of Control, Ross Inst. Tropical Hygiene, Calcuta.*

Idem., (1942) *Ibid.*
Idem., (1943) *Ibid.*
Idem., (1944) *Ibid.*

Ramsay, G. C., Chandra, S. N. and Lamprell, B. A., (1936) *Rec. Mal. Surv. Ind.*, 6, 49-52.

Robertson, J. C., (1910) *An enquiry into malaria in Saharanpur City*, Government Press, Allahabad.

Roy, D. N., (1931) *Ind. J. Med. Res.* 19, 617-628.

Idem., (1939) *J. Mal. Inst. Ind.* 2, 239-242.

Roy, D. N. and Biswas, T.C., (1942) *Ibid*, 4, 417-420.

Russell, P. F. and Rao, T. R., (1940) *Ibid.*, 3, 543-562.

Russell, P. F. and Jacob, V. P., (1939) *Ibid.*. 2, 131-152.

Senior White, R., (1937) *Rec. Mal. Surv. Ind.* 7, 47-75.

Idem,, (1941) *J. Mal. Inst.*, 4, 57-62.
Idem., (1943) *Ibid.*, 5, 207-231.

Senior White, R. and Adhikari, A. K., (1940) *Ibid.*, 3, 383-411.

Senior White, R. and Rao, J. V., (1943) *Ibid.*, 5, 187-205.

Strickland, C., (1929) *Ind. J. Med. Res.*, 17, 174-182.

Strickland, C.. Choudhury, K. C. and Choudhury, H.P., (1933) *Ibid.*, 15, 67-89.

Sur, S. N. and Sur, P., (1929) *Report of Bengal Fish Research Krishnagar Laboratory*, 1926-28, Govt. Press. Calcutta.

Sweet, W. C., and Rao, B. A., (1937) *Ind. Med. Gaz.*, 72 665-674.

Timbers, H. G., (1935) *Rec. Mal. Surv. Ind.* 5, 345-370.

Venhuis, W. G., (1941) *Geneesk Tij. Ned.-Ind.*, 81, 2178-2188.

Vishwanathan, D. K. and Rao, T. R., (1943) *J. Mal. Inst. Ind.* 5, 255-260.

4

Some Important Factors Relating to the Prevalence of Malaria

Continued existence of malaria depends on a variety of factors, chief of them being :

Distribution and prevalence of malaria
Climate
Plant life and malaria
Immunity—race, age, sex and occupation
Man-made malaria

Distribution and Prevalence

Malaria is a focal global disease, and extends to 60°N latitude in Russia and 40°S in Argentina; as high as 9000 feet in Quito in Ecuador and as low as 1300 feet below the sea in the Dead Sea. The distribution of malaria in the world is usually divided in three zones, *viz.*, the temperate zone (40°N to about 60°N with patchy distribution of malaria and benign tertian as predominant species and with little malaria in the corresponding zone of the southern hemisphere), the subtropical zone (Tropic of Cancer to 40°N and corresponding zone of the southern hemisphere, with autumnal epidemics and malignant tertian as the common infection and benign tertian frequent in the malarious regions) and the tropical zone (Tropic of

Cancer to Tropic of Capricorn with malignant tertian are predominating parasite, wide distribution of the disease and in areas near the equator throughout the year). The Indian subcontinent with its greatest length north to south about 2000 miles and its greatest breadth from east to west about 1500 miles, shows a very great variation of physical features. In the wide range of its latitude and longitude it offers an Arctic climate in the snow-clad areas 15000 feet up in the Himalayas and a great belt of temperate and tropical climate lower down. The winter isotherm at the foot of the Himalayas is about 50°F. The plains of the north have extremes of climate, bitterly cold in winter and blistering hot in summer. The south remains hot throughout the year (winter 75°F., summer 80°F.). Rainfall varies from place to place, from the world's highest record of about 430 inches at Cherrapunji in Assam to less than 6 inches in a year in Rajputana and the west. The greater part of the Punjab (pre-partition) contains rich alluvial soil, brought down by the rivers, while the southern tableland is composed of rocks with a thin layer of soil. The western parts of India and Malwa have black cotton soil. The Assam Valley between the Burma Hills and the Himalayas is 50 miles wide and 300 miles long and is full of detritus to a depth of about 3 miles. The melting snow from the Himalayas gives rise to a 7 miles wide river, the Brahmaputra. Heat and moisture help thick forests like those of the Sunderbans to flourish at the mouth of the Ganges, whereas heat with no moisture pervades the deserts in Rajputana and the west. Depending on the fertility of the soil, the population in the Indo-Gangetic plains and on the Western and Eastern Coasts is very thick, but in Sind and Rajputana sparse. These widely different conditions of soil and climate, varying from snow-bound rocks to warm well-watered and fertile valley, persuade men to sow different crops by different methods, to undertake different irrigation and engineering projects. They provide breeding places for different species of anopheline mosquitoes.

Knowles *et al.* (1930) observe that zoographically the Indian sub-continent differs from other malarious countries at all points except as regards the North East Frontier. The

Persian desert cuts it off from the malarial region of Mesopotamia in the west, the Pamirs separate it on the north west from the malaria of the lower Oxus Valley whilst to the north the Himalayas and the immense tableland of Tibet, at an elevation inhibitory to the disease, separate it from the malaria and is known to occur in Siberia. With the exception of the North East Frontier, the ocean bounds the remainder. It must have been through the corridor of the Brahmaputra-Yangtse that malaria entered the country. Kashmir, which is the farthest point from the entrance, is comparatively malaria-free. *Plasmodium malaria*, the species which produces the smallest absolute number of gametocytes (owing to the fact that its schizonts only produce some 8 or 9 merozoites from some of which gametocytes result) has not yet reached the west of India to any extent.

The following is the general trend of the malaria season in India :

Assam	March to June with a peak in May-June. Second wave of fresh infections from September to November with a peak in October.
Central India & Indo-Gangetic plain	July to November with a peak in September. Second wave of B.T. relapses and delayed primary infection in April and May.
Foot-hills	February to June.
Plains	Autumn or early spring.
Southern India	Depends on the terrain and rainfall.

The Public Health Commissioner in his preliminary Annual Report for 1939 states :

"Areas 5,000 feet above sea level area are non-malarious and four widely separated regions, *viz.*, Eastern Bengal, the North-eastern portion of Brahmaputra Valley in Assam and two narrow strips of territory in Madras Presidency, in the Northern Circars and around Madras City, are relatively free from the disease, the spleen rate being under 10 per cent. The malarious tracts can be divided into five main types representing varying degrees of prevalence of the disease. The first consists mainly of the coastal regions of the maritime provinces of Bombay, Madras and Orissa, of wide areas in the Gangetic Valley, of the United Provinces (Uttar Pradesh) and Bihar and of large tracts in the Central Provinces (Madhya Pradesh) and the eastern portion of Central India. In these areas malaria is prevalent in a more or less static form of moderate to high endemicity, fulminant epidemics being uncommon. Another type of malarious region exhibits the hyperendemicity associated with jungly hill tracts and foothill areas. These areas are widely scattered in the sub-Himalayan regions of the United Provinces and Bengal bordering on Nepal and Bhutan respectively, in Assam, the Chittagong Hill Tracts, the Central Provinces, the Chhota Nagpur Hills and in the Western Ghats. A third type consists of an extensive tract of dry area running across India from north to south and comprises Sind, Rajputana, the south-western portion of the United Provinces, a large part of Central India, Gujarat, Bombay, Deccan, Hyderabad and Mysore States and an area in Madras Presidency to the east and south-east of Mysore. This region has varying degree of malarial endemicity depending on local factors such as irrigation. There is usually an autumnal rise in fever incidence and epidemics of malaria may take place at intervals of a few years. To the north of this large area lies a territory consisting of a considerable part of the Punjab, Delhi Province and the north-western portion of the United Provinces, the boundary running well to the east of Agra and Bareilly. This region is liable to outbreaks of fulminant epidemics of malaria, the spleen rate being high during and immediately after such epidemics and slowly falling to a low rate in the course of five or six years. A fifth type showing hyperendemicity unassociated with hilly conditions exists in strictly localised areas, for example, the Tanjore District of Madras Presidency, a thin coastal strip above Madras City and isolated spots in Orissa and Bengal".*

*See page 43.

Climate

Temperature, rainfall and humidity and sub-soil water level etc., in a locality have a direct bearing on the prevalence and seasonal distribution of malaria. Gill reported from the Punjab that when the mean monthly temperature and humidity fell below 61°F. (16°C) and 63 per cent respectively malaria was not transmitted. A favourable temperature and humidity may prolong the life of a mosquito. Atmospheric conditions in a place may not be suitable for anopheline breeding places or the development of sporogony cycle in the mosquito. Rainfall may give rise to numerous breeding places in one area, whereas it may wash the larvae down the hill streams in another. Mosquitoes can live with difficulty in high temperature with low humidity and at low temperatures they do not bite. They can, however, live for long periods with infected blood meal and can convey the disease when the temperature rises again except when they are in a state of complete hibernation. With high humidity the mosquitoes may not only live to allow the parasite cycle to be completed but to transmit the infection to several persons. The minimum temperatures for continuous development of *P. malariae*, *P. vivax* and *P. falciparum* are generally 16.5°C., 17.5°C. and 18°C. respectively.

Plant Life and Malaria

Plants provide under certain circumstances protection and food to mosquito larvae. In *jheels*, tanks, ponds and numerous collections of water, a careful observer will find four different zones of vegetation. A bottom zone (vital layer) of silt with microscopic plants, putrefaction bacteria, sulphur bacteria, iron bacteria, unicellular plants (the Diatoms) and blue-green algae ; the second zone of flowering acquatic plants rooted to the bottom layer (*viz*., ribbon-shaped green leaves with underground trailing stems of the *Vallisneria spiralis*). The third zone is composed of floating and submerged vegetation. The commonest water plants in India are the *Hydrilla verticillata*, *Ceratophyllum demersum*, *Myriophyllum tuberculatum*, *Lagarosiphon Roxburghii*, *Najas indica*, *N. foveolata*, *Utricularia flexuosa*, *U. stellaris* and others. Finally the fourth zone is composed of numerous floating and amphibious plants. The floating vegetation may be non-flowering water plants or minute flowering plants like Wolffia, Lemna and Azolla (which incidentally serve as food for fish). But often these non-flowering or minute flowering plants are replaced by larger plants such as *Pistia stratiotes, Salvinia cucullata* and water hyacinth. These large plants provide support to various types of amphibious vegetation like *Jussiaea repens, Ipomoea reptans, Enhydra fluctuans* and *Hygrorhiza, aristata*, etc. The vegetation, if allowed to grow unchecked, forms a dense canopy on the surface of the water. The activity of the putrefying bacteria and Schizomycetes of the vital layer converts rotten vegetation and organic matter into nutrient salts, and provides inexhaustible food for the growth of plants. Dense vegetation consequently develops and puts an end to the life of various fresh aquatic fauna like cyclops, copepods, rotifers, paramecium, amoeba and other lower members of the animal kingdom. (These smaller members form food for crustaceans, fish, etc.). The adverse effect on the various fauna is mainly due to absence of light and oxygen and the presence of gases. The association of various types of vegetation with breeding places of various species of mosquitoes has not yet been throughly investigated, but there is no doubt that further researches will soon establish intimate relation of various species of mosquito with different types of aquatic growth. Reference has been made (while discussing bionomics of the different species) to the fact that breeding places of *A. philippinensis larvae* are associated with *Hydrilla verticillata, Cerctophyllum demersum, Utricularia, Najas* and non-holding masses of filamentous green algae. Duckweed, water hyacinth, blue-green algae such as *Anabaena, Oscillatoria, Mycrocystis aerugenosa* and *Euglena* and other flagellates appear to render the collections of water unsuitable for breeding places of *A. philippinensis* larvae. *A. sundaicus* is often associated with vegetation such as algae (*Enteromorpha, Cladophora, Cynophyceae*), *Oscillatoria germinata, Lyngbya Confervoids Oedogonium* and dead aquatic vegetation (*Potomogenton pectinatus, Halophilaovata* and the well known brackish water blue-green algae *Lyngbya aestuarii*). *A. annularis* like *A. philippinensis* is found associated with floating vegetation composed of *Hydrilla verticillata, Ceratophyllum demersum* and algae growth, mainly of *spi-*

rogyra. *A ramsayi* is found occurring with *Pisita stratiotes* (Biswas, 1940, 1944, 1945).

Immunity

It is common experience that some patients suffering from malaria spontaneously recover without any form of specific treatment. Spontaneous recovery of the patient infected with malaria parasites points to a very efficient defence mechanism in the body. Experiments on rhesus monkeys infected with *P. cynomolgi* and *P. knowlesi* show that defence against malaria, as evidenced by the death of parasites during acute rise of *P. cynomolgi* or *P. knowlesi* infections (natural immunity), or by the increased death and destruction of parasites during and after the crises of *P. cynomolgi* infections (acquired immunity), is essentially a local immunity in strategically placed organs. Phagocytic activity, lymphoid hyperplasia and the concomitant cytogenesis of macrophages are initiated in the spleen, and are always most pronounced in this organ. As the intensity of malarial stimulation increases, these changes also occur, though to a lesser degree, in the liver, and to an even lesser extent in the bone marrow (Taliaferro and Mulligan, 1937). Neurosyphilis cases receiving repeated malaria parasite inoculations during their treatment become refractory to the same strain of malaria parasite. West Africans are reported to have acquired a high degree of immunity to local strain of malignant tertain malaria. It appears that each dose of parasite injected into the body gives tolerance to the strain of parasite injected. The immunity to local strains starts developing from childhood and youth as a result of repeated attacks of malaria. In highly malarious areas infant mortality therefore is verh high. The individual remains immune provided he continues to be re-inoculated by the mosquito with a local strain of parasite practically throughout the year, or at least for 8 months in the year. Even then the protection or immunity is not absolute. The protective armour breaks under the strain of injury, fatigue, exposure, under-nourishment, and changes with altitude.

Ethnic Groups

The difference noted in different groups in India is probably due to difference in acquired immunity and facilities of personal protection from mosquito bite (screened houses, mosquito nets, clothing, etc.) and antimalaria measures taken.

Age

In hyperendemic areas, every infant is likely to be infected soon after birth. Spleen and parasite rates amongst such children will be obviously higher than amongst adults. In moderately endemic or relatively healthy areas, adults may show higher parasite and spleen rate than children for the simple reason that, as a person grows, the chances of his being bitten by an infective vector increase.

Sex

Women in India are probably more exposed to bites of mosquitoes, as they remain in the house for the most part of the day, and are usually working both in the early hours of the morning and late hours in the evening. Congenital malaria very rarely occurs as a result of transfer of parasite from the maternal blood to the foetal blood through a tear in the placenta. Menstruation appears to have no relation to the frequency or severity of the infection.

Occupation

Aggregation of labour, movement of labour from one locality to another in malarious surroundings, occupations in which men are employed at night, or in those where any or all the various factors giving rise to malaria are present, will have a great influence on the incidence of malaria.

Man-made Malaria

The human hand has played an important part in creating, inadvertently, breeding places for mosquitoes ; and has consequently helped in spreading malaria. Pits all over the urban and rural areas, burrow-pits along roads, railways, quarries and engineering projects are not infrequent sights. Embankments interferring with the natural flow of water and promoting water-logging have provided ideal breeding places for mosquitoes. Large irrigation projects, where necessary precautions have not been taken, have not only increased the cultivable land but also the menace of malaria. The Sukkur Barrage and Mettur Irrigation Projects are well-known examples.

Regional epidemic have flared up where there was large aggregation of labour and ill-advised modification to natural surroundings were carried out. The hill section of the Bengal Assam Railway is an outstanding example where jungles were cut down and graves took their places. It is stated that one man died for every sleeper laid.

Malaria Forecast

For malaria to spread, there must be infected persons with sufficient number of malaria parasites, female anopheline mosquitoes with facilities to breed and bite human beings and the presence of susceptible individuals. Epidemics occur when a large number of non-immune persons enter into a locality, or if a foreign strain of malaria parasite is introduced into a community. In areas where reinoculation, practically throughout the year, does not take place, seasonal epidemics occur if there is an increase of the infective vector with facilities for spread of infection. The Punjab (pre-partition) Health Department used to forecast the probable incidence of malaria every year in the beginning of September. The method of forecasting was based on the hypothesis that malaria epidemics occur due to the loss of equilibrium between infection and immunity, consequently involving the consideration of humidity, spleen rates, epidemic potential and economic factors. An excessive rainfall in July and August, extensive floods, a relatively high epidemic potential factor (above 60), a low spleen rate in June and a famine or relatively higher price during the preceding year. give warning of the onset of an epidemic. Such forecasts, based on the above mentioned factors, have proved of immense value to warn in good time the areas likely to be affected. (Butt, 1944).

Epidemics

The sequence of events in epidemics may be summarised

as follows. The surviving malaria carrying mosquitoes lay eggs. By the end of a week or ten days adult mosquitoes emerge. They may take blood fed from human beings who are gametocyte carriers. The number of such carriers, however, is low at this stage. The few female anopheline with infected blood feed are able to infect other human beings by about the end of third week. A few cases of malaria thus occur by the end of the fifth week. The persons now infected produce large number of gametocytes by the end of the sixth week and infect many mosquitoes. The infected female anophelines in their turn are able to infect many persons by the end of the eighth week. Thus by the end of the tenth week from the initial laying of eggs an outbreak of large number of malaria cases occurs. The subsequent events depend on the conditions favourable for propagation and longevity of the carrier species, communal immunity and facilities for the spread of infection.

From the above very brief account, the complexity of the malaria problem is obvious. The principal factors not only differ between districts of the same State but also in rural and urban localities of the same district. The same species of mosquito may behave differently under different conditions, *viz. A. maculatus*, a dangerous vector in Malaya is relatively innocuous in India. *A. philippinensis* is found in human habitations in Bengal, but rests in cattle sheds in Assam. It is probable that these are biologically distinct races of the same species. Strains of malaria parasites show a wide variation. A community may be relatively immune to a particular strain of a species of malaria parasite and show a very low incidence of malaria, but a foreign strain may precipitate an epidemic, if circumstances are favourable for the spread of infection. It is essential to study and make a survey of each locality before attributing incidence of malaria to any of the factors referred to above. Different species of anophelines may require different control measures. It is easy to understand how immense harm can be done by putting embankments, railways, roads, drains and barrages in places where from malaria point of view, they are not desirable, by selecting a site for habitation without a previous malaria survey of the locality, by leaving burrow-pits and brickfields unattended thereby increasing breeding places for mosquitoes, by faulty methods of irrigation, by injudicious house construction, by imperfect drainage or sewage system and by uncontrolled aggregation of a large population.

*The Stratification Committee Report (1987) give seven stratums, *viz.*, (*i*) Non-refractory areas with low to moderate epidemic potential, *i.e.*, large portion of South India; (*ii*) Moderately refractory area with high epidemic potential in Central Western India ; (*iii*) Non-refractory areas with moderate to high epidemic potential in Western India ; (*iv*) Non-refractory areas with high epidemic potential in Nornh-Western India, Jammu, Punjab, Haryana, Himachal Pradesh and adjoining areas of Uttar Pradesh except Eastern strip. Western Himalayan Zone including the Sivaliks and the Ganga alluvium ; (*v*) Non-refractory areas with limited epidemic potential in Northern and Eastern India ; (*vi*) Refractory areas with high receptivity malariogenic potential in Central-Eastern and Eastern India ; and (*vi'*) Refractory areas with high receptivity in North-Eastern India.

5

Elimination of Breeding Places

Effective anti-malaria measures include measures to prevent infective species of mosquitoes from breeding, offensive campaign against mosquitoes in all stages of development, careful defensive action to protect human beings from the bite of mosquito, and administration of drugs to kill the parasite injected into the system by mosquitoes that survive offensive action and penetrate defences.

Man-made breeding places in fields and firetins, burrow-pits and brickfields, tubs and tanks, roads, railways and the like, and those in nature like swamps, seepages, etc., can be readily eliminated by simply ensuring adequate drainage of water and by preventing water from collecting.

Swamps and Seepages

Rain water either flows down the earth as surface water and runs in streams, rivers and ultimately into the sea, or percolates into the earth, emerging lower down as seepages and swamps. Uusually some of it runs as surface water and the remainder sinks into the earth. Such collections of water can be got rid of by a well planned system of drainage. The drainage may be open on the surface or subsoil, leading from subsidiary drains to the main drain.

Surface or open drains should be narrow, with sides free from vegetation, and with adequate fall and depth and rounded bottom. Subsidiary drains or tributaries should join it at an acute angle. In swamps they can be made to run parallel or in herring-bone arrangement. In foot-hills it is best to mark out soon after a shower of rain, areas of highest springs and seepages, and then to dig a contour drain of adequate size (usually 4′ deep, 6′ wide at the top and 1′ at the bottom) at right angles to the flow of water down the foot-hill. Excavated earth should be thrown at least 10′ behind the drain. Drains have been excavated in the U.S.A. and Palestine by laying dynamite charges 1½ feet apart in holes (Svensson). This method has been found not only labour saving but also quick. The drains may be built with or without lining. *Pukka* cement or stone is not absolutely necessary for more than 3″ above the normal flowing water level in the drain. If the storm-water drain is intended to carry sullage in addition to rain water, the whole drain should be lined and provided with central cunette for carrying the perennial flow, giving the least breeding surface. The unlined drains often get damaged and require constant attention in cleaning and grading. These drains can also be made of circular pipes 4″ to 12″ in diameter, 1′ to -′ long, or open concrete inverts can be laid and covered with gravel and earth and thus prevent rain from damaging the top. The laying out of sub-soil drains requires skilled labour. Initial cost is high but recurring expense is low. They can be easily supervised.

Faggot or fascine drains have been successfully used in Malaya and Africa (Watson, 1942) on a large scale. Drains are filled with lengths of cut bamboos complete with leaves as they are cut from the trees. In a mine in Africa, these covered drains were made in 1932 and were found working well for long periods up to 1939 without any repairs or upkeep. Stone packed drains can also be made. They often require renewal. Sub-drainage has been used in Kangra Valley and has turned a highly malarious water logged area into a cattle grazing ground free from malaria (Raina, 1946). All that was done was to dig *kutcha* surface drains ; they were covered with flat stones and earth, and grass was planted on top.

At times it is difficult to drain collections of water lying over an impervious stratum. In some cases a pit can be dug and a shaft driven vertically down through the impermeable stratum. Stones are packed roun ; the shaft. These vertical drains in selected suitable places effectively accelerate percolation of water. The number of such vertical drains, depends on the size of the area to be drained. In a few cases all that is required is to submerge or to flood the swamps by putting weir lower down. These can be sluiced, or larvae can be dealt with by a suitable antilarval method. Invariably the rule of "decreasing the inlet or increasing the outlet" helps to get rid of the collection of water. It is, however, emphasised that it is not necessary to drain all pools and swamps, if larvae are not found breeding in them. Injudicious construction of drains in areas where the vector mosquito breeds in running streams is obviously dangerous In some areas with moderate monsoon rainfall bunds are put so that rain water is directed to a single Lido or depression.

Burrow-Pits and Brickfields

It is a common practice to dig earth for the construction of roads, railways, canals, embankments and in brick-kiln areas, leaving behind vast pits below the drainage level. If the earth so excavated as to leave an even slope, no water will collect. Where such a procedure is not possible, the pits can be dug in series, connected with each other and sloped so that no water is able to accumulate. Partial filling may be required in places to ensure a proper gradient. A note of warning may again be given that draining of the pits by connecting them can lead to dangerous breeding places in areas where the infective vector breeds in drains with grassy edges and running water. In such areas it may, be possible to break the impervious stratum and make vertical drains. Filling in of pits is ideal but the cost is often prohibitive.

Quarries

Quarries leave numerous depressions. Quarrying should be done vertically so that the face is only very slightly undermined (preferably not at all undermined), leaving no chance for water to collect.

Holes in Trees, Rocks and Sand

Holes in trees and rocks require filling with earth. Crab holes and the like may be filled with Paris green sand or earth.

Fields

Fields with wet cultivation may be associated (especially in the case of irrigation channels in the rice fields) with malaria. Fields flooded with silt are less liable to breed mosquitoes. The incidence of malaria may depend on the methods of irrigation. Perennial irrigation channels from canals give rise to seepages and water-logging, and inundation irrigation leaves pools after the flood subsides. Counter-drainage, good maintenance of channels and sluice gates, and restrictions on water supply can reduce the number of breeding places considerably. Channel banks should be protected if necessary by fencing. Disused water courses should be filled in as far as possible. Intermittent drying of fields reported by Russel has proved a great success in South India, where rice fields are kept dried for two days in the week. Kalandadze and Sagatelova (1944) have drawn attention to the fact that anopheline eggs or larvae may not die unless drying is absolutely complete, as in the presence of slight moisture the eggs, especially anopheline eggs, can survive for over a week. Intermittent flooding has not only reduced the number of breeding places but has in many cases improved the yield of crops.

Pipes

Piped water supply for irrigation or domestic use requires constant supervision of hydrants, storage tanks and stand pipes. Hydrants and sluice valves should not leak. A concrete platform with a proper drain to allow the water to run off should be provided round hydrants and stand pipes.

Wells, Tanks and Swimming Pools

Wells can be rendered innocuous by introducing larvivorous

fish, or sealing the top with concrete and lifting the water by means of a pump. A mosquito-proof cast iron inspection door can be incorporated in the concrete seal.

All water cisterns similarly require well fitting lids and side holes must be closed in all cases to prevent entry of mosquitoes.

Water in the swimming pools, etc., should be changed weekly.

Drains

Domestic and sewage drains require special attention. As far as possible they should not cross the road or neighbouring houses. They can be made of semi-cylindrical glazed pipes or concrete halves. The terminal drains can be rendered mosquito-proof by covering the last 75′ with concrete. If the connection is made with a pipe of 6″ diameter, a 12 feet "off set" effectively prevents the entering of mosquitoes and consequently prevents breeding. The same principle holds good for ventilation shafts. Ventilation shafts of dimensions of more than 6″ diameter will require mosquito-proofing. The main drains are usually 8′ wide at the top, 2′ at the bottom and 5′ deep.

Sewage Disposal

Sewage disposal (except when in the sea or large rivers) requires constant supervision. *A. stephensi* has been reported to breed in sewage contaminated water.

Roads and Railways

Embankments put across natural drainage lead to the rise of subsoil water and obstruct the flow of storm water, and thus lead to numerous collections of water. All embankments across the natural line of drainage should be avoided. Drains should be provided on either side of the embankments, so that any water likely to collect is drained off. In road and railway construction, the problem of embankments requires serious consideration. A sufficient number of bridges and culverts with inverts placed at correct level can prevent collections of water. Collections of water on roads built under bridges may require pumping out.

Dams and Barrages

Dams and barrages often give rise to a number of breeding places. Drainage of overflow, prevention of leaks and provision for rapidly lowering the level of water in impounded waters, help considerably in reducing mosquito breeding.

Jungle Clearance

Indiscriminate clearing of jungle is dangerous. Bionomics of the mosquitoes should be studied.

Dry Day

There are numerous breeding places that can be eliminated by every individual. Pots and pans, tins and bottles should not be carelessly thrown away. Small collections of water in pits and pools, in and around houses, should be filled or drained. It should form a rule in every home to empty all vessels containing water like *chatties*, buckets, etc., at least once a week. In public institutions like schools, offices and municipalities, a *dry day* every week should be observed. The object of this measure is that on one day in the week every place is kept completely dry for a short time. A thorough inspection of the whole area within fixed hours should be carried out to ensure that no collection of water has been overlooked.

REFERENCES

Covell, G,, (1941) *Anti-mosquito measures* with special reference to India. Health Bulletin No. 11. Malaria Bureau No. 3, Manager Publication, Delhi.

Kalandadze, L. P. and Sagatelova, (1944) *Trop. Dis. Bull.* 41, 916.

Raina, B. L., (1946) *Anti-malaria measures Yol., Kangra Valley*, (not published).

Svensson, R. *A handbook of malaria control*, Shell Book Oil Companies.

Watson, M, (1942) *Some Emergency Anti-Malarial Measures*, Ross Institute Industrial Advisory Committee, 6.

6

Anti-Larval Measures

Before starting anti-larval measures it is necessary to study the local breeding places, the ecology of the mosquitoes, particularly the vector species. Much time, labour and money can be saved if those places only are treated which breed mosquitoes, especially the vector species. It may be added that in an area, other species of mosquito though not responsible for carrying malaria, have great nuisance value, especially during the spring in the plains, and their breeding should also be controlled. The areas to be controlled will depend on various factors, including species of anopheline mosquito, the nature of the breeding places, the prevailing wind, distance of human habitation from the breeding place, etc. It may be stated as a general rule that control over an area up to at least half a mile round an inhabited locality gives satisfactory results. Ribbands (1944) however points out that the risk of getting infection is negligible if five miles, and is small if two miles, intervene belween the camp and any infected locality. Risk of getting infection however increases if there are breeding places between the infected area and the area to be protected or the number of residents in the locality is small. Raevsky and his colleagues (1944) have reduced the risk by putting cowsheds and animal houses on the leeward side between the breeding places and human habitation (mosquitoes start feeding on cattle instead of men). The animal sheds are put not less than

200 meters from the human habitation (piggeries 250 m.). The animal houses should be separated from each other by following gaps: byres 50 meters, pigsties 45 meters, sheep pens 50 meters apart with doors on the leeward side. There should be vegetation between the barrier and human dwelling. Cattle must return from grazing not later than half an hour before sunset.

Anti-larval measures wherever feasible should be permanent. Temporary measures invariable prove expensive in the long run due to the recurring expenditure.

Temporary measures, however, will be required in many places during the construction of works, collection of large number of people for a short period and during the interim period when permanent measures are being made.

Anti-larval measures can also be naturalistic or chemical.*

Naturalistic

Naturalistic or biological measures aim at so altering the natural conditions as to render the place unsuitable for breeding. The following methods have been successfully, used against larvae of different species :

Sluicing, flooding, silting, agitating the surface of water, changing its level, etc.

Deep shading.
Pollution.
Changing the salt content.
Alteration of food supply.
Larvivorous fish.

Sluicing : The sluicing is only an imitation of nature's method of flushing down the larvae; water of a stream is dammed and released at intervals by either hand-operated sluice gates or by automatic siphons. Sluice gates were first used

*The dangers of pollution of food by chemical larvicides and insecticides are now well recognised. Great caution in their use has to be observed. Naturalistic or biological measures have no such dangers.

by Graham at Lucknow at 1913 in the river Gumti. They were popularised as malaria control measure by Prof. K. B. Wiliamson who used them between 1930-32 in Malaya against *A. maculatus*. By 1937 about 200 streams along 15 miles of

Automatic Flushing Siphon De Villier's Type

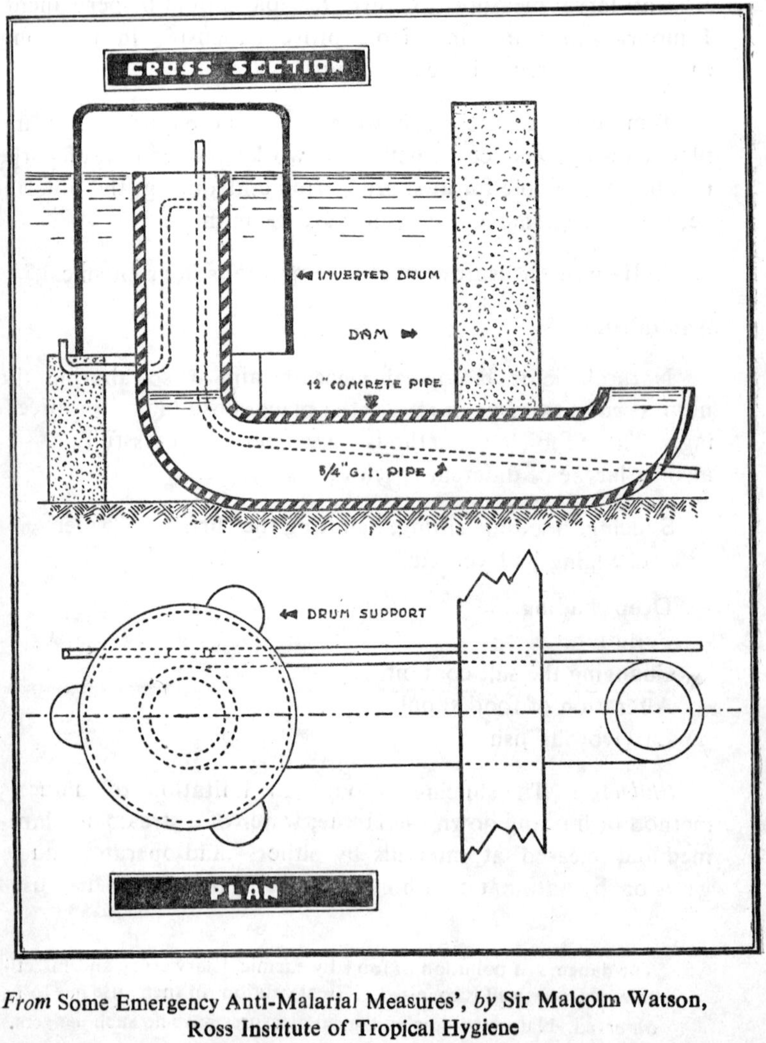

From Some Emergency Anti-Malarial Measures', *by* Sir Malcolm Watson, Ross Institute of Tropical Hygiene

hills in Penang were being successfully flushed. By the force and disturbance of water, larvae are washed down and stranded. In some cases eggs and pupae drift to the banks lower down and require further treatment. Macdonald designed an automatic siphon incorporating DeVillier's siphon with full flush of 475 gallons per minute at a cost of Rs. 25 per siphon. The main parts of DeVillier's siphon are an inverted oil drum on three concrete blocks, a main siphon made of concrete or earthen-were pipe which runs under the dam and a secondary siphon consisting of 3/4″ galvanised iron pipe.

In small streams, earth dams with one or more oil drums, the ends of which had been removed to form an opening through the dam for releasing the flush, have been used in South India. The upper end of the drum is kept closed by a sheet of wood until the dam is full, then the wood is removed by hand and the stream is flushed. Various other sluice gates (like drums fixed eccentrically so that they tilt immediately they are filled up with water and resume vertical position when empty) have been improvised at a very low cost (Watson, 1942).

The pipeless siphon used in Tea Estates is a great improvement. The principle on which they work is that when the water rises in the catchment area, it flows over the weir and falls into the sealing trough below at the outflow taking air with it. When water falls in the trough, some of these bubbles come up on the outside of the trough, thereby causing a partial vacuum inside the siphon. This unequal pressure between the outside and the inside of the siphon starts the flow of water expelling all the air inside the siphon. When the water level in the catchment area falls sufficiently low to admit air to enter at the inlet, the vacuum is removed and the siphon immediately shuts off until the water level rises and the cycle again commences. Atmospheric balancing valves are placed at the highest point of the siphon, so that, by opening these valves, the siphon may be stopped at any stage of working (Ramsay, 1944). These siphon may be of any size and shape, depending on the quantity of water to be released. Water released must not exceed the amount normally carried in the channel during floods. Like all measures sluicing has its limitations. Site and distance between the series of sluice gates in a stream will vary with different places.

Automatic Pipeless Siphon

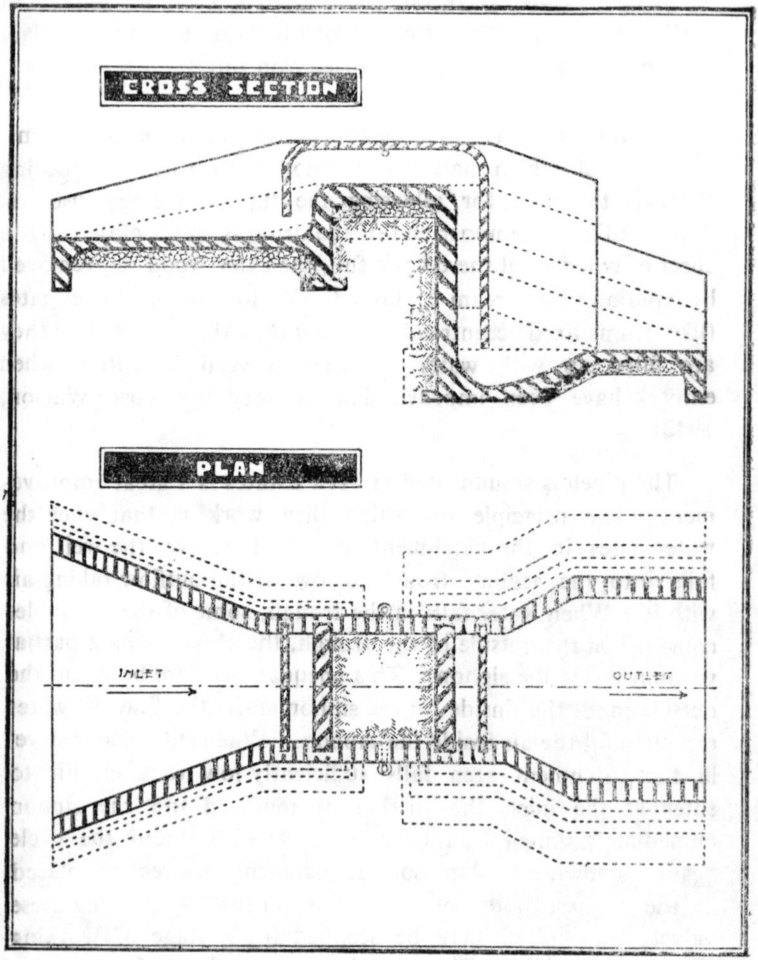

Courtesy Dr. G.C. Ramsay

Flooding : Floods with silty water have been noticed to reduce the incidence of malaria. Rise of water level in Bengal is a good example. Sinha (1940) gives seven reasons in favour of a flood flush scheme, *viz.*, it maintains during the rainy season flow of silty water in the drains; ditches, water channels, pools burrow-pits and low lying areas as a result of which mosquito breeding is easily and effectively checked. The low-lying areas, small pits and depressions are gradually filled up by silt deposit. It helps local drainage by discharging water when the tide is low. It feeds numerous tanks and ponds with good river water and thereby improves the water supply. It introduces millions of fish, spawn and fry, which not only destroy the mosquito larvae but also augment the fish supply of the rural areas. Not only does it lessen the malaria incidence by preventing mosquito breeding, but it also improves the agriculture of the land by depositing silt over the cultivated plots, which have a high maintenance ; hence such schemes are economically very sound. Bentley recommends that the canals should be run full during the flood season to flood the largest possible area with silt-laden water.

Fluctuation of water : Fluctuation of water and agitation of the surface of water have been used very successfully in ponds, lakes, marshes and impounded waters, particularly in the T.V.A. in the U.S.A.

Deep shading : Dense shading has been used for a long time in Tea Estates to combat breeding of *A. minimus*. Dense shade keeps the edges of the streams clear of grass and weeds, and thus eliminates the common sheltering places for the mosquito larvae. Dharanta, eupatorium bougainvillia or bahok and lantana have been used in various places. The best examples of shading in low-lying swampy lands are reported to be in Balisera Valley, Sylhet District, and Assam. When planting hedges, it is important to raise the bank of the drains well above the flood level and high enough to enable the hedge to establish itself (Ramsay, 1942). The hedge takes about two years to grow. Places where it is likely to be damaged by cattle require fencing. Shading to be successful should be dense throughout the controlled channels, as any break in the shade will provide breeding places for the anopheline larvae. 'Beehive' or 'pent-house' pruning of hedges is reported to produce maximum foliage (Ramsay, 1944a).

Pollution of water : Dirty, black, offensive collections of water are still considered by many to be breeding places for mosquitoes, but brief notes on bionomics of the dangerous vectors in India given in the previous section show that majority of them breed in fresh and clean water. Pollution of water with cow-dung, effluent from sewage works, factories. soap water, cut vegetation and herbage packing have been used with varying degree of success. Mosquitoes may breed, but the dangerous anopheline mosquitoes can be easily eliminated at a comparatively low cost. Pollution with rusty water containing iron oxide deprives larvae of algae and has been reported favourably.

Salt content : Brackish water provides breeding places for *A. sundaicus.* It has been effectively dealt with by changing (increasing or decreasing) the salt content of the water.

Alteration of food supply : In Java, by emptying and drying of the fish ponds, green algae were replaced by blue green algae, which provided neither shelter nor food for the larvae of *A. sundaicus.*

Larvivorous fish : Several species of fish have been used to free tanks and pools from mosquito larvae. Seal and Moore carried out valuable investigations under the United States Fish Commission. Many years ago Ross noted that certain fish feed on mosquito larvae. Numerous workers have confirmed the utility of larvivorous fish in India. The top minnow (*Gambusia*) extensively used in Italy, South America and West Indies, and imported into India about 1929 from Italy and Siam, has established its reputation as a valuable naturalistic control measure. Three imported and about twenty-two indigenous fish have so far been described as larvivorous. The three exotic are fairly well known, *viz.*, Gold fish (*Carassius auratus*), the popular ornamental fish imported from the Far

East, Barbados millions (*Lebistes reticulatus*) used in Ceylon, which was imported into India but could not be acclimatised here, and the top minnow (*Gambusia affinis*) the most extensively used fish and distributed free by the various fisheries and anti-malaria centres. Hora and Mukerji recommended the following in order of larvivorous activity: Top Minnow, *Panchax*, *Aplocheilus*, *Aphanous*, *Carprinus* (*Puntius*), *Osphranemus* (*Colisa* and *macropodus*). Favourable reports have been received about the larvivorous activity of *Haplochilus*, *Barbus*, *Chela Barilius*, *Ambassis nama*, *Trichogaster fasciatus* and *Schizothorax progastus** (Raina, 1944).

Widely divergent views are held regarding the utility of indigenous fish. Hacket pointed out that "the local fish after centuries reach a balance regarding their natural enemies, and the number cannot be artificially increased and maintained at an abnormally high level of density; whereas, if exotic fish can be acclimatised, they will proliferate and maintain their number at abnormally high level". On the other hand Fry Hora, Prasad, Sweetnam and Meyers advocate the use of indigenous fish and condemn the use of exotic fish on biological grounds. There is enough evidence to believe that some indigenous fish

*For effective biological control of larvae by fish, it is essential to know the bionomics of the mosquito and ecology and biology of the fish. The importance of fish in malaria control has been established for a long time, but the habits of the various indigenous fish have not been scientifically studied in detail, and have not been tried on a large scale in the field. To prove conclusively the part that fish play as larvivorous agents and to determine the utility of various indigenous species, Prasad and Hora (1936) suggested that as a preliminary measure two adjoining areas, one heavily infested with malaria and the other comparatively free from it, should be selected for survey. An intensive survey of the fish fauna of the two localities should be undertaken, due regard being paid to any correlation that may exist between the probable density of population of the mosquito larvae in the different areas of the locality, and the types of fish and density of their population in the same kinds of water. Observations should also be made of the natural food of various types of fish by an examination of their stomachs.

like *Panchax*, *Aplocheilus*, *Aphanous* and *Schizothorax progastus* are equally larvivorous as exotic genera.

Larvivorous fish have their limitations. In temporary, collections of water or in places used as permanent fisheries, their use is not recommended. Prasad and Hora suggest that "for fish to be effective all vegetable matter and debris that may prevent access of fish to mosquito larvae should be removed. This means that areas of water to be treated should be kept clean and in as much sanitary condition as possible : (*a*) all predatory fish should be removed ; (*b*) disconnected pieces of water separated by short distances, such as burrow-pits etc., should be connected by a regular drainage system so as to enable the fish to wander everywhere ; (*c*) shallow pits and pools should be either filled up or deepened, so that fish may be able to live in them even when the water is at its lowest level in the dry weather ; and (*d*) fishing should be strictly prohibited in such areas". Covell enumerates the following requirements (based on Chaudhury's paper) for useful larvivorous fish :

"They must be small so that they can get about in the shallow water among weed, etc.

They must be hardy and flourish both in deep and shallow water.

They must be able to breed freely in confined water areas.

They must be able to stand transport and handling.

They must be difficult to catch and able to escape their natural enemies including man.

They must be absolutely worthless and insignificant as food.

They must be top-feeders and carnivorous".

Gambusia satisfies the above conditions and is at present readily available from the Malaria Institute of India Delhi.*

Chemical

Oil, Paris green, pyrethrum : Oils, Paris green, pyrethrum and DDT are common larvicides. Cuprous cyanide has also been used and found to be satisfactory as a larvicide under certain climatic conditions. Paraformaldehyde, soap, cresol, commercial Cyllin, creozote, carbolic acid and borax have been used as larvicides, but are not in use now. Nesterwodskaja and Lubinski (1944) have reported that phenothiazine (7 and 14 ounces per acre at 12-13°C.) kills all mosquito larvae in 48 hours.**

Oiling : L. O. Howard in 1892 first recommended oils as larvicide, and suggested that the film of oil mechanically stops the breathing of mosquito larvae. The larvae are killed not only by suffocation but also due to irritant and toxic action of oil mixtures. Sir Malcolm Watson showed that mosquito breeding can be stopped even in running water by spraying the

*There is a strong case for use of indigenous larvicidal fish, on biological grounds. They donot disturb the ecological balance and propagate freely in their natural habitat *Schizothorax progastus* is a good illustration. At the time of its discovery as a larvicidal fish in 1944, its size and quality of being good for eating were considered as enough reasons to reject its use. One encouraging note was from Sir Malcolm Watson. In his letter of December 1945 to Raina, he observed : "Perhaps if enough grew, there would be enough both for food and to kill larvae". Despite general criticism, the water holes, streams in Yol were stocked with the fish. It was easy to collect from the places where they were locally found in plenty and distribute to other places. After five years Lt. Colonel K.S. Pillai. Executive Medical officer Military Hospital Yol in his letter of October 1949 states : "*Schizothorax progastus* are progressing quite well ; there are also in some parts of streams including Nod khud; they are thriving in Tanda near Kangra. Bowlees and streams with *Schizothorax progastus* are completely free from mosquitoes larvae ; the results of experiments carried out to test their larvicidal qualities, as compared to *Gambusia affinis* are quite satisfactory".

**Recently other larvicidal agents have been used. Temephos at a dose of 1 ppm at intermittent intervals of two months or more is reported to be very effective against *A. culicifacies* breeding places stream, its banks and seepages with oil, and pointed out that what is sold as crude oil or fuel oil varies greatly in composition in different parts of the world, and that many of these oils do not make satisfactory anti-malaria mixtures. Some would not kill larvae, some would not destory the grass, some would not spread, some require admixture of economical amounts of kerosene and some were quite useless. G. Watson (1941) carried out a series of experiments to demonstrate the action of various oils and oil mixtures on larvae, and reported that the time available for killing the mosquito larvae is the time until they next moult their skin. If, before this happens, enough oil enters their trachea to obstruct moulting or suffocate them, if their skeletal muscles are paralysed even by momentary contact with oil or if their food supply is poisoned so that they starve to death, then the oil mixture and the method of applying it, have been successful. It is obvious that, before using any oil or suggesting any oil mixture, it should be seen that it satisfies the above conditions. Expensive oils are not necessarily good larvicides. Highly refined oils often lose their toxicity.

Oil used as a larvicide should have a spreading pressure of at least 23 dynes/cm. Dyne is the term used to express the force of the oil film which overcomes the resistance to its spread. The commonly used oils have spreading pressure of about 23 dynes/cm. Larvae in water with dense vegetation require oils with spreading pressure of 46 dynes/cm. Kerosene has usually 10 dyne/cm. Gas oils have 13 to 16 dynes spreading pressure. Addition of cresylic acid 0.25 per cent to 1.5 per cent commercial resin greatly increases the spreading pressure.

The Burmah-Shell Oil Company, in close collaboration with the Ross Institute of Tropical Hygiene introduced malariol, which is being widely used as a mosquito larvicide. It is highly toxic to larvae, pupae and eggs. It has good spreading power and burns vegetation. A suitable mixture can be made from the available oil in a locality, like waste engine oil mixed with kerosene, or malariol or Attock malaria oil, by actual experiments in the laboratory and the field, Macdonald recommends a film not less than 10 microns thick, *i.e.*, 14 gallons of malariol per acre or 3 gallons per 1000 sq. feet. Fifteen to twenty-five gallons per acre, 1½ ounce per square yard, in practice have been used with very good results. One to two gallons of oil per 250 yards may be required in streams. Oiling preferably, should be done against the stream. The sprayer should be kept about one foot above the water level. Vegetation on the bank should be cleared before oiling is done. High pressure sprayers kept in good repair are very satisfactory. Oiling once a week is as a rule satisfactory. The water used for drinking and in fields should not be oiled, as this will render the water unsuitable for drinking and will burn the crops. Wells and drinking water can be successfully treated with petrol at 24 oz. per 80 sq. ft. of water surface; if alowed contact for two or three hours, it rapidly kills the larvae. Oiling in irrigation channels 400 ft. short of fields has been tried without any harm to the crops. It is necessary to avoid oiling irrigation channels in close vicinity to fields, where, if the edges are kept clear of grass, one can usually effectively control mosquito breeding.

Oil drip cans are not recommended except in norrow channels, as the dripping oil flows down the middle of the stream, and does not affect the grassy edges. In broader streams one drip can on either side near the edge will be useful. Oil booms have been used with success to treat larval drifts, *i.e.*, larvae carried down into protected areas from outside. Methods suitable for local conditions can be improvised. In certain main streams gunny bag screens soaked in oil, overlapping at the edges and placed at intervals of 100 yards, have been used with success. Saw dust, rice husk or *bhusi* soaked in oil and thrown in the collection of water after the manner of sowing seeds proves very effective.

Oil is very useful as a temporary measure in temporary collections of water or during the period when permanent measures are being taken. In lakes, rivers and streams, etc., oiling the grassy edges alone has given good results.

Paris green : Barber and Hayne carried out experiments with various arsenical compounds, and reported that copper-aceto-arsenite (Paris green) is a powerful larvicide. Good Paris green contains 56.6% of arsenic as arsenious oxide. For Paris green to be effective it should contain over 50 per cent arsenious oxide The usual strength of Paris green used is from 2½ per cent to 5 per cent (1 per cent when dusted by hand, 5 per cent when dusted with blowers, 75 to 33 per cent by aircraft have been used). Metcalf and Hess report that *Anopheles quadrimaculatus* larvae can ingest particles of 29, 51, 68 and 106 microns in 1st, 2nd, 3rd and 4th instars respectively. De Andre reports that best results are obtained with Paris green 2 microns in diameter. The only guiding factor for the necessary strength of Paris green to be used is a practical test in the field. If a particular strength is not found effective, it should be increased. Numerous substances have been used as diluents. The commonly used diluents in India are ash, screened road dust, sand, slaked lime, soap stone powder, cement dust and saw dust. For large areas like streams, heavy diluents are often suggested. The diluents should be passed through a screener before use. The vehicle and the Paris green used are thoroughly mixed in the required proportion generally in a rectangular galvanised iron box supported on two pillars. The mixture is dusted usually with hand bellows or rotary blowers. Paris green has been sprayed with success from aeroplanes—one pound of Paris green per acre is usually required. Paris green may also be applied in liquid form. Since Barber used the Paris green solution in Greece, Russell and Jacob (1939) and other workers have used it successfully in India. A stock mixture of kerosene oil ½ gallon, Paris green 2½ lbs., castor oil 1 oz., and white of 4·6 eggs, shaken up in a pint of water can be used. This mixture in dilution of 1 oz. to 1 gallon of water can be used in a sprayer. Paris green mixed with water (in dilution 1 in 500 or 1 in 250 suspension) has also been used (dose one gallon to 870 sq. ft.) effectively in shallow streams.

Dusting and spraying with Paris green is a cheap anti-larval method, and is specially suitable for fields and irrigation channels. Frequency of dusting depends on intensity of breeding and the climate. If the development of the larvae takes less than a week or so, application every fifth day may be necessary ; in other cases application once a week gives quite good results. It must be remembered that Paris green has no effect on eggs or pupae of mosquitoes and does not kill culicine larvae, when applied in the usual method. The use of Paris green has almost now been replaced by DDT.

Dichlor-Diphenyl-Trichlorethane (*DDT*). Its chemical synthesis was done as early as 1874 by a German chemist from Strassbourg. In 1939 a firm in Switzerland (J.R. Geigy Company) during investigation for moth killing agents came across this chemical. They promptly produced it under the name "Gesarol". In 1942 the New York Branch of Geigy Company received 200 lbs. of DDT from Switzerland. The Department of Agriculture in Washington immediately got it from New York Branch of Geigy Company and forwarded it to Orlando Laboratories. It was soon found to have insecticidal properties against body lice. In January 1943, chemists of the United States Department of Agiculture at Boltsville, Maryland Laboratories identified it as Dichlor-Diphenyl-Trichlorethane. Following its identification, intensive research both in the field and the laboratories was taken up by British, American, Indian and other workers. In a short time it struck a death blow to insects carrying diseases in various theatres of war. It was soon found to be lethal to mosquitoes, lice, flies, bugs and various other insects.

DDT is a white crystalline powder, nearly insoluble in water, moderately soluble in petroleum and vegetable oils and readily soluble in most organic solvents. It has 1.6 G per millilitre density. Crude commercial forms vary in purity and may contain only 60 to 77 per cent pure DDT (para para or p'p' DDT). p'p' DDT melts at 108°-9°C. It has a characteristic and pleasant odour and a tendency to clump. Exposure to high temperature and humidity increases its tendency to clump. It is toxic to most crustacea and insects. Ellis *et. al.* (1944) report that gold fish weighing 6-10 G die after taking pellets of DDT 63-200 mgm. per kgm. body-weight and frogs died after 40 to 72 hours on a single parenteral dose of 150 mg.

per kgm. Rats and guineapigs after absorption of DDT through the skin showed toxic necrosis of the liver and kidneys. The lethal does for animals varies from 150 to 600 mgm. per kgm.

Solubility in common solvents in per cent p'p' DDT at 27-30 C is as follows :

Toluene	...	...	... 38
Veg. Turpentine		...	... 20
Malariol	...	...	... 9
Fuel Oil (Diosel) No. 2			... 9
Fuel Oil (Diesel) No. 1			... 7
Kerosene Crude		...	... 7
Kerosene refined		...	... 4

Solution of required strength can be easily made by breaking up the lumps of DDT and then making a paste with the solvent. It can then be poured into the container. The container should at least be ¼ full of solvent. Finally the remaining solvent is poured in the containers. The solution in the container is kept in the sun and stirred with a stick (or by bubbling air with a power driven air compressor). The solution is ready for use in 3 days. For immediate use DDT can be heated slowly on a hot plate and poured into the solvent when molten, stirring all the time. A 3.7 per cent solution can be conveniently made as follows : A four gallon tin is filled with commercial DDT up to 3½" from the top. This approximates 22.5 lbs. of DDT. Assuming that the powder contains 75 per cent of p'p' DDT when it is dissolved in 45 gallons of the solvent, the resultant solution approximates 3.7 per cent solution of p'p' DDT.

Its effect on eggs and pupae is negligible but is lethal to larvae and adult mosquitoes.

DDT as larvicide. It is interesting to note that there is selective absorption of DDT on the chitin *in vitro.* Its larvicidal action is due to ingestion of the chemical or absorption or both.

As a control measure 0.15 lbs. (2.4 oz.) of p′p′ DDT per acre is found satisfactory. DDT-malariol solution gives better results than DDT kerosene mixture. It is observed that 0.3 lb. DDT per acre kills fish, frogs, snakes and other acquatic animal life. Care, therefore, is required not to exceed the strength of DDT in water used for breeding of fish. The following have been used successfully :

(*a*) 7 ounces of DDT to 1 gallon of 3rd quality kerosene oil resulting in a 5% solution. One quart of this solution is sufficient for one acre.

(*b*) 0.1 lb. DDT per acre, in thick vegetation up to 1 lb. per acre for dusting.

(*c*) 2½ per cent to 3.7 per cent DDT solution in kerosene oil with approximate dosage of 0.15 lbs. of DDT spraying with Kent type pneumatic knapsack sprayer per acre.

(*d*) Five per cent DDT solution in kerosene oil in a bamboo stump with one end of bamboo plastered with mud thrown in the middle of the pond. Dosage 0.2 lbs. per acre.

(*e*) One handful of 2 per cent DDT powder mixture five pounds per acre.

(*f*) Sand or step bricks soaked in DDT thrown in stagnant water.

(*g*) 3.7 per cent DDT solution mixed with dry sand and made into balls thrown at intervals across water surface. Balls made with mud are found ineffective.

Even one to two quarts of 5 per cent DDT solution per acre have been found effective.

The opinion is gaining ground that discrete application is preferable. Five per cent solution in an oil of 46 dynes/cm. spreading pressure gives good results on still waters. Two ounces should kill all larvae within 25 feet radius, *i.e.*, about 2000 sq. feet. DDT in emulsified solution have also given very good results.

Whatever the method used, one must ensure that the breeding surface is completely covered. In every case, care should be taken to distribute DDT uniformly, especially along the water edge. If spraying is done intermittently, the intervals should not exceed 5 yards. The density of vegetation and scum modify the effect for obvious reasons. Pouring by hand, or garden syringes, dusting or throwing sand and bricks are not so effective and economical as spraying with knapsack sprayer or stirrup pump. In South East Asia Command, during the war DDT was extensively sprayed from aircraft. 0.3 to 0.6 lbs. DDT per acre is usually effective. 5 per cent solution of DDT were used singly or in formation flights with several aircrafts abreast. The dosage of 2 to 3 quarts per acre of the solution controlled mosquito breeding in swamps. Full destruction of mosquito breeding in streams covered with vegetation was not possible. The DDT deposited on vegetation, however, killed the mosquitoes coming to lay eggs and those which were newly hatched. Application of DDT by aircraft has since been developed to a high degree several types of aircrafts including helicopters with various types of equipment are now employed.*

REFERENCES

Ellis, M.M., Westfall, B.A., and Ellis M.D. (1944) *Science*, Nov. 24, 477.

Hora, S.L. and Mukerjee. *Table for identification of some Indian fresh water fish*, Manager Publication, Delhi.

Nesterivadskaja, K.M., Labiniski, G. A. (1944) *Tr. Dis. Bull.*, 41, 103.

Prasad B., and Hora, S. L., (1936) *Rec. Mal. Surv. Ind.* 8, 631-46.

Raevsky, G. E., (1944) *Tr. Dis. Bull.*, 41, 543.

*Evidence is accumulating on harmful effects of insecticides and pesticides on human beings. This requires constant review on their use.

Raina, B. L., (1945) *I. M. G.*, VLXXX, 273.

Ramsay, G. C., (1942) *Report of the Committee of Control, The Ross Institute of Tropical Hygiene, India Branch.*

Idem (1944a), *Ibid.*

Idem (1944b) *Personnel Communication* forwarding a note by J. Robertson.

Ribbands, C. R., (1944) *J. Roy, Army Medical Corps.*, 82, 157-64.

Russell P.F. and Jacab, V.P. (1939) *Jl. Mal. Inst. Ind.*, 2, 261-271.

Sinha, J.D., (1940) *Bengal Public Health Journal*, II, 23.

Watson, G., (1941) *Bull. Ent. Res.*, 31, Part 4.

Watson, M., (1942) *Some Emergency Anti-malaria Measures.* Ross Institute Industrial Advisory Committee.

7

Anti-Mosquito Measures

Various methods of killing the mosquito have been used, *viz.* trapping, swatting, fumigating with sulphur dioxide, cresol, lysol, Izal, chlorine gas, etc. and spraying with pyrethrum, DDT, BHC. An effective, practical and popular method at present is spraying with DDT or pyrethrum or DDT mixture.*

Pyrethrum : Le Prince and James in 19 6, Ross in 1936 and Meillon in 1936, Covell, Mulligan and Afridi in 1938 reported remarkable results by spraying pyrethrum solution. One part of 2 per cent pyrethrum extract in 19 parts of third grade kerosene oil was recommended. A very effective spray can be prepared by soaking one pound of dried powdered pyrethrum flowers in one gallon of kerosene oil for 72 hours, provided the flowers are of good quality (Covell, 1941). Many proprietary products containing pyrethrum extracts are now available which are equally effective. It is essential not only to spray the affected locality but also all buildings within about half a mile

*Malathion is also a popular method. It is reported to have brought done the malaria incidence (where anti-larval measures against *A. culicifacies* were ineffective) when indoor residual malathion spray in the peripheral areas was combined with space spray with pyrethrum.

Among the recent anti-mosquito spray, good reports have been recieved of Pirimiphos methyl.

around it. The spraying must be done thoroughly and systematically. It is necessary to close all doors and windows, open up all cupboards and almirahs, etc. (if any), and start spraying with the spray directed upwards. Direct hits on mosquitoes need not be aimed at. Pyrethrum is a contact poison, and its lethal action is most pronounced in atomised cloud. The spraying in the room or hut should be continued till sufficient concentration of the solution is produced (causing very slight irritation to the eyes). The quantity recommended is 1 oz. of spray per 1000 c. fit. of space. The room should be left closed for about half an hour, after the spraying. The uninhabited huts or houses, etc. should not be neglected. It is best to plan out a definite circuit for each set of houses. Thorough spraying will be required in most places in the early morning not later than one hour after sunrise.

The principle of adult spraying is that malaria can only be transmitted by the female anopheline mosquito, which, having fed on a person with gametocytes in his blood, succeeds in surviving for at least 10 days and then has the opportunity of bitting another susceptible human being. The object is not so much to prevent human beings from being bitten by the mosquito as to reduce the longevity of the carrier species to such an extent {that it cannot live long enough to become infective and as such cannot transmit malaria.

A very simple hand sprayer (MISH pattern) has been designed by the Malaria Institute of India. Excellent results are obtained with petrol driven paint sprayers. Electric sprayers of the same pattern are equally useful. The American aerosol bomb is a great improvement over the hand sprayers. All that is required is to unscrew the cap over the nozzle of the bomb. Immediately after the removal of the cap a fine mist containing the insecticide fills the room. Sesame oil acts as an activator of pyrethrum enhancing its insecticidal properties, and Freon 12 (dichlorodi-fluormethane) acts as the propellant providing the necessary pressure to expel the insecticide. About 4 seconds are required to spray a space of 1000 cubic feet. Each "bomb" can effectively kill all flies and mosquitoes in 100.000

cubic feet. DDT with an auxiliary solvent is now added to pyrethrum—Freon 12 solution.

DDT : The DDT is absorbed through the tarsi of adult mosquitoes and in a few hours the insect becomes inactive. It gets tremors due to the neurotoxic poison and dies. If the dose of DDT is small and contact time short, the death may take 12 to 24 hours. During the contact and the time of death it often shows increased activity and is not usually found near the place where it had the fatal contact. The dry powder has no repellent action on the mosquito A 5 per cent solution of DDT is 3rd grade kerosene oil is often used. For killing adult mosquitoes optimum results may be obtained with 85 mgm. p'p' DDT per sq. ft., *i.e.* one quart of 3.7 per cent pp DDT solution per 500 sq. ft. With residual deposits of 100 to 200 mgm. p'p' DDT per sq. ft. the residual fatal contact effect can be prolonged. The residual effect is shortened on surfaces exposed to sunlight and rain, porous and painted surfaces. The residual effect has been reported to last several weeks and months.*

Barrier spraying. It was observed during trial in the Fourteenth Army (Afridi) that spraying of a site and a belt of 50 yards round it including buildings on the inside and the outside and every feature in the terrain with 5 per cent DDT in kerosene oil at the rate of 5 gallons per acre prevented 90 per cent of prevailing mosquitoes from infiltrating into the protected zone. Spraying of a 50 feet belt only round a camp site was not so effective as in the case where camp site itself was sprayed. Area and zone spraying requires repeated spraying after 10 days and therefore this method can be used only if the stay in a place is of short duration.

Residual spraying should be started in and around the

*Some vectors (*A. culicifacies, A. stephensi, A. annularis*) were reported as resistant to DDT, dieldrin and malathion in a number of places in the country. In some places the vector resistance is to a single insecticide, in others to two or three insecticides and in still another (*A. stephensi*) varying degrees of resistance to a number of insecticides.

buildings one month before transmission of malaria is due to commence and repeated monthly throughout the malaria season. If it is found that the infective mosquito rests on the exterior of the building after taking its blood feed, the exterior of the building should also be sprayed. The spraying should be done so as to deposit effectively DDT crystals in the required strength on all the surfaces where the mosquitoes are likely to rest. It is done effectively with the Four Oaks pattern knapsack sprayer or stirrup pump with special nozzle. The minimum dosage of solution which can be applied evenly from distance of one foot from the wall in the case of Four Oaks sprayer is one quart per 250 sq. ft. The stirrup pump with the same quantity can spray up to 500 sq. feet. By increasing the distance of the nozzle from the wall the dosage of solution can be decreased. Although the stirrup pump requires two persons to operate and its rubber tubings sometimes burst during spraying, it can effectively spray with a speed of 4 feet per second without contaminating the clothes of the operator to a considerable degree. A few precautions are essential during spraying. No food, cooking utensils, etc. should be allowed to be contaminated with DDT. The persons employed to spray should use protective eye shields, gloves and overalls while spraying and should have a bath with soap and hot water after spraying.

Other Insecticides : A lot of experimental work has been done lately to alter DDT molecule and also to change the number of chlorine atoms in DDT molecules to substitute other chemical groups such as Flouro-Bromo and Methoxy. A number of solvents and emulsifiers have been used.

DDD, DFDT, DMDT and the like are less toxic to human beings and insects. DDD has almost the same or better action than DDT on larvae but is less toxic to adult mosquitoes. By completely altering the structure powerful insecticides like benzene hexachloride, chlordane or octachlor, toxaphene or chlorinated camphene and parathion have been produced.

Imperial Chemical Industries, Ltd. has introduced Gammexane which contains the gamma isomer of benzene hexachloride. 6.5 per cent of this isomer is present in Gammexane powder P520. Ross Institute of Tropical Hygiene recommend a single dose of 10 mg. gamma benzene hexachloride per square foot to obtain control of adult anopheles for a period of at least three months. Twelve ounces of Gammexane P520 mixed with one gallon of water and dispersed at the rate of half a gallon per 1000 sq. ft. give a deposit of about 11 mg. gamma B.H.C. (gamma isomer) per square foot.

Chlordane has been widely used with success in Italy against house flies. Toxaphene has the same residual toxicity as benzene hexachloride and chlordane. High toxic effect is also claimed for 497 and 118 but sufficient data are not yet available to give any definite opinion. Hexaethyl tetraphosphate, tetraethyl pyrophosphate and diethylnitro phenyl thiophosphate (parathion) are other insecticides belonging to phosphate series. It, however, has not prolonged residual effect but is effective against immature stages of insects. In the phosphate series parathion is the most important.*

Synergists

Work is also being carried out on synergists for DDT. Synergists can be put in two categories, *viz.*, those affecting physical properties of the residual deposit and those which are toxic in themselves. Gum rosin 10% is often used. Gum rosin acts as nuclei for DDT crystals. They not only tend to increase the toxicity of the DDT but the adhesive property of gum rosin prolongs their residual action. The common examples of toxic complementary synergist are of pyrethrum and DDT, methoxychlor and DDT and chlordane and DDT.

It may be emphasised that the use of modern insecticides like DDT as a residual spray has proved that it is the most effective and practical method of controlling malaria, especially

*Recent practices include malathion fogging/ULV spraying during epidemic of Japanese encephalitis/malaria contingency measure; spraying of BHC where Japanese encephalitis cases repoted are 100 or more in a year during the past decade.

in rural areas. It is obviously necessary to organise and plan the spraying after carefully considering the ecology of the local mosquitoes, especially the local vector and investigating local conditions.

Love call trap. Reference may be made to an interesting experiment carried out by Kahn *et al.* (1945). They have found that mosquitoes make various sounds while flying and by beating wings or rubbing tarsi against wings. These sounds include a 'love call'. On hearing 'the love call' (audible and inaudible to human ear) of a single female mosquito, numerous male mosquitoes turn their antennae and hypopygium towards the female and burst into a chorus. Work is being continued to produce the love call mechanically in DDT treated spots in the hope that all made mosquitoes within hearing distance will come into the trap and die. This would avoid spraying of large areas with DDT.

Personal protection. Personal protection from mosquito bites by suitable house construction. Use of nets, suitable clothing and repellents are still some of the effective methods of preventing malaria infection.

House construction. Screening of buildings in malarious localities is of great value. The following figures by Hanif as early as 1928, showing the result of screening in British troop barracks in Lahore, speak for themselves :—

Year	Admission per 1000 screened barracks	Unscreened
1926	182.1	572
1927	45.6	265.9

The main objection to screening often put forward is that the atmosphere inside screened houses is suffocating and the rooms become dark. Lack of light and ventilation is often noticeable in houses which were originally built on the usual popular plans, and of which the screening of doors and windows is done afterwards. Covell (1941) recommends that the following principles should be observed, "Building to be screened must be built and kept in good repair. Door frames should be made of seasoned wood with iron brackets at the corner, and should not sag on their hinge. A double wire attached diagonally across the lower half of the door and tightened up with turn buckle will tend to prevent this. No attempt at edge fitting should be made. The door should be made to fit against a $\frac{3}{4}''$ batten all round the inside and sufficient space allowed for the door to swell in wet weather without scraping at the bottom. A light strip of wood should be nailed across the door frame at about the height of a man's shoulders. This is to push against when opening the door. There should be two fastenings for each door, one half way up the top section and one near the bottom. The lower panel of the door may be strengthened by wire netting as a protection against kicks and against dogs attempting to enter or go out. Doors should open outwards so that mosquitoes resting on them may be driven out when they are opened. They should be placed on the windward side of the house, for the mosquitoes tend to congregate on the leeward side. It is of great advantage to have double doors with a porch or vestibule at least 6 feet in length between them. Strong springs should be fitted to the doors to ensure that they will remain tightly closed when not in use. Every aperture in the building should be screened. No removable screens or shutters should be used. No screening should be used within one foot of the floor because it is liable to be damaged when the floor is scrubbed. No furniture should be placed against screening. Putting wire gauze on existing doors and windows affects the ventilation considerably. Windows should be provided for the ventilation lost. In Federated Malay States, when mosquito-proof houses are built and 16 mesh-wire gauze used, the window area is doubled to make up for the loss in ventilation caused by the gauze. The gauze used in the barracks of British troops in India was 14 mesh and 28-30 SWG, giving an aperture of 0,055 to 0.057.* The ventilation lighting can be improved by

*Where *A. minimus* is the vector as in Assam 16 mesh, 28 ISWG giving aperture of .048 inch is required.

electric lights and fans, and by designing the house especially for screening (screens are mainly put round the verandahs). For screening to be effective the persons living in it should not remain out of the house after sunset and before sunrise.

The estimated cost of mosquito-proofing a building in normal times is about 2 to 3 per cent of the total cost of building. Temporary labour camps can be made mosquito-proof by the use of condemned mosquito nets on doors and windows.

Nets. The mosquito netting with a mesh of 28 to 29 holes in a square inch and made of 30/40 cotton will keep mosquitoes out. Nets should be preferably white rectangular in shape with netting also in the roof and no openings inside. They should be set down before sunset. The free border should be tucked in continuously all round the bedding. No portion of it should be allowed to flap about loosely. When going to bed only the minimum portion of the net should be lifted to enter, and then it should be carefully tucked in again under the bedding. Nets should be turned inside out preferably daily, and the pole corners searched for mosquitoes.

Protective clothing. People should wear long sleeve shirts, slacks or *pyjamas* or *shalwars*. The *dhoti* does not give the necessary protection. Mosquito boots or Wellington boots are very useful. In any case every attempt should be made to so clothe oneself that the minimum amount of body is laid bare for mosquitoes to bite. Veils and gloves have been used in various armies for guards on duty.

Repellent. Plain citronella oil applied 3-hourly gives satisfactory results, while naphthalene conc. ext. of pyrethrum cream gives almost the same results. A non-greasy vanishing cream can be made of gum tragacanth powder 2 parts, oil citronella 2 parts, pyrethrum 2 per cent ; 80 parts water is added after mixing all the ingredients. The cream should be liberally applied at 2-hourly intervals on all exposed parts of the body. Dimethyl-phthalate and dibutylphthalate in liquid form are agreeable to use and are very effective, especially the former even when a few drops are rubbed on exposed parts and have replaced the creams used formerly. Its effect !asts for about 4 hours.

D.M.P. fish nets. Afridi *et al* (1945) report that 3/8 inch mesh nets (fish nets), and garments impregnated with 0.42 c.c. dimethyl-phthalate give complete protection from mosquito bites for 72 hours. Nets treated again conferred protection for longer periods.

REFERENCES

Afridi, M.K. and Arthur, J.H., (1945) *South Africa Med. J.*, 19, 361-365.

Covell, G., (1941) *Malaria Control by Anti-mosquito measures*, Thacker, Spink and Co. (1933) Ltd., Calcutta.

Covell, G., (1941) *Anti-mosquito Measures*, Health Bulletin No. II, Manager Publication, Delhi.

Kahn, M.C., Celestin, W. and Offenhauser, W., (1945) *Science*, March 30, 335-6.

8

Malaria Survey & Anti-Malaria Campaign

It will be obvious from the foregoing account that, before starting an anti-malaria campaign in an area, it is essential to carry out a preliminary survey. The survey should include the study of physiographical features, meteorological records, mortality and morbidity by age groups, directly or indirectly, due to malaria, total death and birth rates by age groups in different parts of the year, spleen rate* and parasite rate amongst the children of the locality (children between two and ten years are most suitable for the purpose), seasonal prevalence of malaria, species of anopheline, their breeding places, flora and fauna of the breeding places, bionomics of the mosquitoes and investigation regarding the carrier species. Dissection of gland and gut of mosquitoes with a view to determine the

*Infection with malaria gives rise to enlargement of spleen. The areas are classified usually as follows : Over 50% spleen rate hyperendemicity, 25-50% high endemnicity, 10-25% low or moderate endemicity, under 10% healthy. After 10 years of age immunity starts and by about 15 years of age spleen may become normal. Spleen rate, therefore, is taken of children between 2-10 years.

infection rate and further investigations in detail regarding the bionomics of the local mosquitoes, especially the vector species, will have to be continued as a preliminary survey. Study of social and economic condition of the people and industrial and agricultural problems should not be overlooked.

After deciding the measures to be adopted in a locality it will be necessary to plan a scheme incorporating permanent and temporary measures, and undertake further investigations of the antimalaria problems of the locality. In practice it is useful to divide large areas into small self-contained units. It is the small units which carry out the most important work in the field and are responsible for control measures in a locality. Under a unit scheme, the area of malaria control should include areas ½ to 1 mile beyond the periphery of a locality to be protected. The whole area is divided into sub-areas under a malaria inspector. Each sub-area may be further divided into six zones. The work is so arranged that a field squad works in one zone at a time in rotation, so that each such zone is thoroughly treated at least once a week. It is necessary to keep records of the work done. The following diaries are suggested :*

(1) METEOROLOGICAL RECORD

Year			Month		
Date	Maximum Temperature	Minimum Temperature	Relative humidity Morning Evening	Rainfall	Prevailing wind

(Records must be made at specified fixed times daily. Records of sub-soil water may also be kept if possible).

*With regard to details of malaria survey reference should be made to Health Bulletin No. 14, Malaria Bureau No. 6 and *How to do Malaria Survey*.

(2) MOSQUITO CATCHES

Date				Month		Year
Species	Number	Cattle sheds	Houses	Number from each Mosquito catching station 1, 2, 3, 4.	Precipittin test	*Dissection Gland Gut*

Various traps have been recommended for catching mosquitoes. A type of trap used with success is a simple wire ring 2½ feet in diameter, over which a black or red cloth skirt is stitched with purse string at both ends. These are hung two feet from the ground. Dark red colour appears to attract mosquitoes. In an experiment carried out with red and black traps, 1147 mosquitoes took shelter in red traps and 772 mosquitoes in black traps (Raina, 1943). A red earthenware *chatti* is almost as good. Traps when used are put in corners of rooms in the catching stations. In actual practice a well trained insect collector can catch more mosquitoes than the traps and most of the field workers have practically given up using traps. Such catches can be of value only if the time, duration and technique of catching mosquitoes are uniform. Usually a large number of catches in a day indicate breeding places nearby for which search can be made. For special investigation further information can be added in the same diary, *viz.* catches during the first, second, third and fourth quarters of night, etc.

(3) LARVAE

Year			Month		Date
Place	Type of breeding place	Quality of water	Flora vegetation	Fauna	Species

One of the Malaria Survey and Control Charts

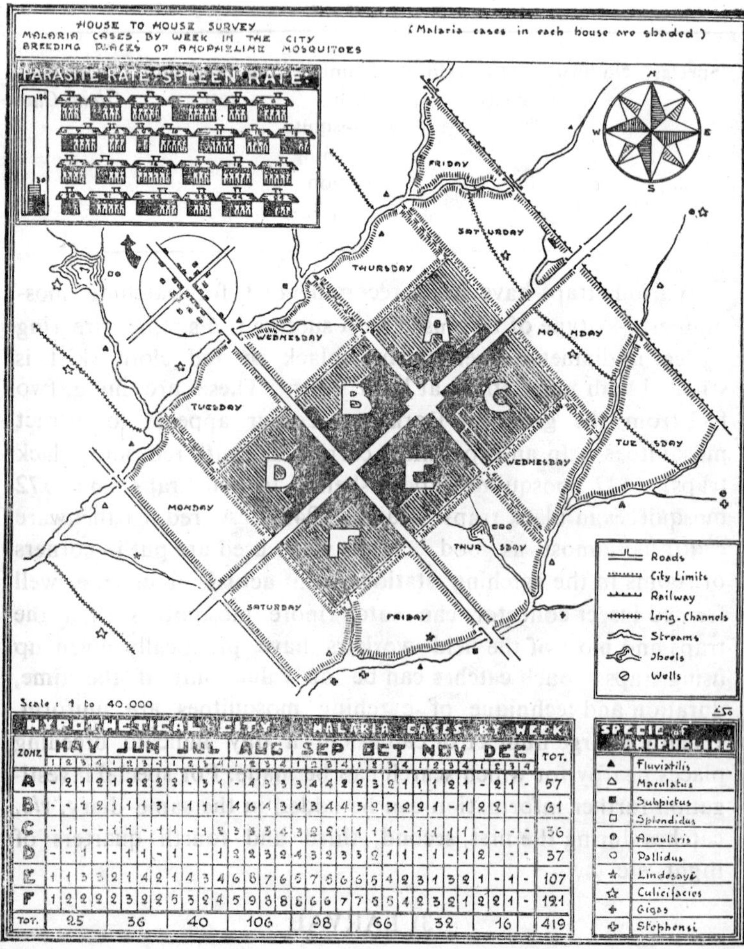

ZONE	MAY 1	MAY 2	MAY 3	MAY 4	JUN 1	JUN 2	JUN 3	JUN 4	JUL 1	JUL 2	JUL 3	JUL 4	AUG 1	AUG 2	AUG 3	AUG 4	SEP 1	SEP 2	SEP 3	SEP 4	OCT 1	OCT 2	OCT 3	OCT 4	NOV 1	NOV 2	NOV 3	NOV 4	DEC 1	DEC 2	DEC 3	DEC 4	TOT.
A	-	2	1	2	1	2	2	2	2	-	3	1	-	4	3	3	3	4	4	2	2	3	2	1	1	1	2	1	-	2	1	-	57
B	-	-	1	2	1	1	1	3	-	1	1	-	4	6	4	3	4	3	4	4	3	2	3	2	2	1	-	1	2	2	-	-	61
C	-	1	-	-	1	1	-	1	1	-	1	2	3	3	3	4	3	2	2	1	1	1	1	-	1	1	1	1	-	-	-	-	36
D	-	-	1	-	-	1	1	-	1	-	-	1	2	2	3	2	4	3	2	3	3	2	1	1	-	1	-	1	2	-	-	-	37
E	1	1	3	3	2	1	4	2	1	4	3	4	6	8	7	6	5	7	5	6	6	5	4	2	3	1	3	2	1	-	1	-	107
F	1	2	2	2	2	3	2	2	5	3	2	4	5	9	8	8	6	6	6	7	7	5	5	4	2	3	2	1	2	2	1	-	121
TOT.	25				36				40				106				98				66				32				16				419

SPECIE of ANOPHELINE	
▲	Fluviatilis
△	Maculatus
■	Subpictus
□	Splendidus
●	Annularis
○	Pallidus
★	Lindesayi
☆	Culicifacies
✚	Gigas
✜	Stephensi

The chart shows parasite and spleen rates in the surrounding villages and area under control, the species of anapheline larvae marked where they are found breeding, area under control divided in six zones A.B.C.D.E.F. and the days on which they are visited by malaria-control sqad and a table showing the number of malaria cases weekly from each zone.

(Labelled specimens should be brought to the Anti-malaria Officer for inspection and verification).

(4) INCIDENCE OF MALARIA BY AREAS
(Zones is possible)

Year	Month	Date

Serial No.	No. of houses	Name S/o	Sex	Age	B.T. Tropho.	B.T. Gm.	M.T. Tropho.	M.T. Gm.	Q Mixed Tropho.	Q Mixed Gm.

B.T.=Benign tertian. M.T.=Malignant sub-tertian.
Q.=Quartan. Tropho=Trophozoites.
Gm.=Gametocytes.

Spleen rate:

Parasite rate:

(5) EXPENDITURE

(6) MEASURES EMPLOYED

The above figures can be consolidated weekly and numbers shown from each zone or barrack, lane or street.

The data so collected can be put down on enlarged maps with different signs, especially showing breeding places (permanent and temporary), mosquito catches, etc. Maps are of great value and show all the facts at a glance. The secret of success lies in good planning, sound supervision, and ability of the organiser to get the work done in the way it should be done.

CHOICE OF CONTROL MEASURES

Measures required for different places will vary. Permanent measures (including biological) should be adopted wherever possible. The former requires a large investment but saves recurrent expenditure except the cost of maintenance. Certain general temporary measures will be always applicable. It has been argued that antilarval measures are conducted in the field and consequently are not easily supervised ; whereas success of antimosquito measure, especially spraying, is easier to organise, easily popularised and gives results in a very short time. Both antilarval and antimosquito measures play an important part in most anti-malaria schemes. The fact that a judicious combination of antimosquito and antilarval measures gives best results is indisputable. Antimosquito measures alone have lately given promising results. The time to start antilarval measures is one month before the malaria season sets in, and the antimosquito measures a fortnight before the onset of the malaria season. If funds do not permit to carry out this procedure, antilarval measures should be started to begin with, and a careful watch kept on the mosquito catches and incidence of malaria. Any rise in a zone in the figures of either or both is a warning that spraying should be started without delay. During the height of the malaria season or when malaria incidence is expected to rise, spraying to kill adult mosquitoes should be augmented. During the non-malarious season measures to kill adult mosquitoes may be suspended. In any antilarval scheme greatest attention must be paid to control species responsible for carrying malaria in a locality, but other mosquito breeding places, including culicine, should not be neglected. Permanent measures including biological should be completed before the malaria season sets in.

REFERENCES

Christopher, S.R., Sinton, J. A., and Covell, G., (1941) *How to do Malaria Survey*, Health Bulletin No. 14, Malaria Burea No. 6, revised by Covell G., Manager of Publications, Delhi.

Raina, B. L., (1943) *Photo Bionomics of Mosquitoes of Kangra Valley* (not published).

9

Chemotherapeutic Agents

Intensive research (pharmacological, chemical and clinical) to find a drug or drugs to ensure a radical cure of malaria has been in progress for many years. Cinchona and quinine held the field for a long time. Since Paul Ehrlich in 1891 reported that methylene blue stains the malaria parasite and is likely to damage it, investigations on synthetic drugs were started leading to the discovery of Plasmoquine by Schuleman and his colleagues in 1924. Mutsche and Mauss carried on the work started by Schuleman and discovered synthetic schizonticide Atebrin in 1930 and Bayers introduced it in the market in 1931. Similar drugs soon appeared in different countries; Acriquinine in USSR, Quinacrine in France, Acridin 10 in India, Mepacrine in England. Since then a number of promising chemotherapeutic agents have been introduced. Many of them are still in an experimental stage. Experiments are being carried out on more scientific basis than before. Not only the action of the drugs on different species of parasites in their different phases (sporozoites pre-and asexual erythrocytic forms, and gametocytes) are investigated but parasiticidal action on different strains of the same species is also observed.

QUININE 6-methoxy-α-(5-vinyl-2-quinuclidyl) 4-quinoline methanol.

Quinine is an effective schizonticide. It is effective against asexual forms of all the parasites. It has hardly any effect on the gametocytes of *P. falciparum*, but destroys effectively gametocytes of *P. vivax* and slowly those of *P. malariae*. Quinine taken by mouth is little absorbed in the stomach and passes through unchanged. Hydrochloric acid of the gastric juice converts insoluble salts into soluble hydrochloride. It is precipitated in the duodenum and absorbed as such. Bile aids in its absorption. Alkalies given before quinine are reported to increase the diffusion through the mucous membrane. The quinine circulating in the blood (concentration usually 1 : 250,000) is taken up by internal organs and split up and destroyed. The remainder is excreted by the kidneys ; excretion begins about ½ hour after taking the quinine and can be detected in urine by Mayer's reagent. Salts requiring preliminary hydrolysis are absorbed slowly. Opinions differ regarding the action of cinchona alkaloids. Morgenroth observed that quinine forms a film on the surface of the red cells and prevents merozoites from entering the cells. Hegner states that the site of action is intra-corpuscular. Bass assumes that quinine renders the cells permeable to blood plasma, so that parasites are destroyed by lysis. Yorke and Macfie suggest that quinine kills some parasites by direct action, while others are killed by the defence cells of the body activated by parasitised products (Field as quoted by Jogleker 1940). Taliaferro (1949) states that "Quinine acts directly on the parasites and may kill them though their death is more commonly the effect of immunity process". Moulder (1950) suggests that quinine 'appears to exert its effects through preventing (the formation of the postulated reactive 2-carbon particle) pyruvate oxidation in the early stages'. Soabra (1950) 'with an ultramicroscope observed that when blood and colloidal quinine solution placed together, the quinine colloidal particles absorbed on the RBC, the degree of absorption depended on the reaction of the blood. If acid absorption was intense, if alkaline it was feeble or absent'.

The usual dose of quinine sulphate is gr. vii to gr. x thrice daily by mouth giving a plasma concentration of 4 to 5 mgm. per litre. In children the dose is usually calculated at 1 to 1½ gr.

plus half the age. In severe cases with hyperpyrexia, hyperparasitaemia or vomiting gr. x of quinine hydrochloride or bihydrochloride in 20 c.c. of 25% glucose solution intravenously given at the rate of 2 c.c. per minute or quinine hydrochloride gr. x (preferably mixed with urethane) in 2 to 4 c.c. of distilled water intramuscularly is usually given.

The Malaria Commission of the League of Nations recommended that the standard product of cinchona should contain not less than 70 per cent of crystallizable alkaloid, of which at least 1/5 should be quinine. This was included in the British Pharmacopoea 1932 as totaquina, which is as effective as quinine. Acton (1920), Acton, Cwajel and Dewy (1921), Prain (1924), Acton and Knowles (1924), Fletcher (1925), Berkely Hill (1926) and James (1927) reported on great value of cinchona febrifuge. Hicks and Dewan Chand (1935) held the view that therapeutically, quinine and totaquine are of equal value. Napier in 1945 made the interesting observation that "the recent work has in no way questioned the efficiency of quinine and other cinchona alkaloids. On the contrary it has confirmed all previous works regarding the antimalarial activity of these alkaloids and more specially of the mixed alkaloid preparations which some of the poorer malarious countries may on economic grounds still prove to be the drug of choice for the mass of population". It may also be added that Mac Gilchrist (1915) working in Calcutta showed that parasite clearance in BT obtained with quinine in 4.7 days, 5.5 with cinchonine, 5 with quinidine and 5.6 with cinchonidine. In MT infection the figures were 6.1, 5.6, 4.85 and 4.3 respectively showing that in BT quinine acts most rapidly while quinidine in MT. Lane quoting Cordes (1924) and Ciuea *et al.* (1925) observed that in MT cinchonine is less satisfactory than quinine and chinconidine was less effective than quinine or cinchona febrifuge respectively. Workers of Medical Research Council of the United Kingdom reported in 1926 that quinine and quinidine are equally effective. Pranger and Filer (1949) have reported that cinchona alkaloids act synergistically with each other in blood induced infection in bird malaria. They also observed that combination of cinchonidine and quinine produce more favourable results than quinine alone in blood induced infection of *P. relictum* and *P. gallinaceum*.

The route of administration of quinine has been a subject of great controversy, particularly the intramuscular injection. Alkaloid injected intramuscularly causes tissue necrosis, which may involve nerves and blood vessels ; in some cases abcess formation occurs and infection with tetanus is possible (if proper aseptic precautions are not taken). Clayton (Lane as quoted by Joglekar *loc cit*) remarks that giving an intramuscular injection is "to push into a patient with a hypodermic syringe a lasting conviction that if it has come to a choice between bitter taste and bitterly painfull experience, it is better to take quinine by the mouth after all." In case of intravenous injection action is rapid (90% passes from circulation within a minute of injection) and without pain. Toxic symptoms are rare if the injection is given slowly.

Although many of the synthetic anti-malarials have been found effective against acute attacks, opinions regarding the prompt use of intravenous quinine in emergency cases like those of cerebral malaria are unanimous (Covell, 1949, Black 1949).*

ATEBRIN (MEPACRINE ; QUINACRINE) 6-chloro-9-(4-diethylamino-l-methylbutylamino)-2-methoxy acridine.

Its, action is more or less like quinine. It is a polyvalent schizonticide. Its effect is more prolonged than that of quinine. It does not destroy the gametocytes of *P: falciparum*. It is extensively localised in the tissues and slowly released. Large loading dose is therefore necessary to build plasma concentration. Headache, restlessness and gastro-intestinal disturbances may be noticed. Yellow staining of the skin may be seen but is transient. The initial loading dose for effective clinical cure

*Intravenous preparation of quinine salts are still considered life saving in cerebral or other serious types of malaria where other drugs fail.

varies from 0.6 g. to 1.0 g. The dosage commonly used is given below :

	1st day	2nd day	Succeeding five days
For partially immune	0.6 g.	0.3 g.	0.3 g.
For non-immune	1.0 g.	0.3 g.	0.3 g.
	or	or	
	0.9 g.	0.6 g.	
	or		
	0.6 g.		

PLASMOQUINE (PAMAQUIN) AND OTHER 8-AMINOQUINOLINES

The action of the plasmoquine group of drugs on schizonts of *P. vivax* and *P. malariae* is considered inferior to quinine, and has hardly any effect on schizonts of *P. falciparum*. On the other hand, it is a polyvalent gametocide, especially a powerful gametocide for *P. falciparum*. It was known as early as 1928 that relapse rate of *P. vivax* under quinine-plasmoquine treatment can be reduced. Herein lies its special advantage. It is relatively a toxic drug. Cynosis due to the formation of methaemoglobin, haemoglobinuria, abdominal pain and vomiting have been often observed, and its routine use is not recommended. Pentaquine and Iscpentaquine in the order stated are less toxic than pamaquine. The dosage usually recommended is 0.06 g. pentaquine base daily with 2.0 g. quinine sulphate for fourteen days. Pentaquine monophosphate contains 75% of the base. The patient should be under hospital observation when taking these drugs for obvious reasons.

CHLOROQUINE DISPHOSPHATE AND RELATED 4-AMINOQUINOLINES

Chloroquine relieves acute attacks of malaria and is a powerful suppressive drug against falciparum infection. Partially immune have been reported to be cured by a single dose of 0.5 g. Like mepacrine plasma concentration is built up slowly unless initial loading dose is given.

It is very active against all asexual erythrocytic forms. Generally clinical cure is obtained in two to four days as against a week with mepacrine treatment. None of the other 4-aminoquinolines (santochine, oxychloroquine, etc.) appear to be superior to chloroquine. The dosage* used in the U.S.A. and Venezuela is as follows :

	1st day	Succeeding days
U. S. A.	1.0 g. divided in two doses	0.5 g. for three days
Venezuela	1.5 g. divided in three doses.	1.5 g. divided in three doses. on second day only.

Camoquin also has been favourably reported.

PROGUANIL (PALUDRINE) N_1=p-chlorophenyl-N_3-isopropyl diguanide.

It is a powerful schizonticide in benign tertian and malignant tertian malaria. Malignant tertian infection can thus be completely cured. It is believed to be the only antimalarial which in non-toxic dosage is a true casual prophylactic against malignant tertian infection. There is wide margin of safety between toxic and therapeutic dose. Paludrine monohydrochloride contains 86.5% of paludrine dose. The usual dose for adults of Paludrine monohydrochloride is 0.3 g. daily for five to ten days. Slight toxic effects like vomiting and renal irritation have been observed. But the toxic symptom disappears on the reduction of dosage or if the drug is stopped for a day or two. It has been recently reported from Africa that attacks of fever resulting from Rhodhsian strain of *P. falciparum* were not controlled for three or four days after paludrine therapy

*For present dosage recommended in India, see pages 90-91.

and attacks of malignant malaria were reported amongst persons who were under paludrine suppressive treatment. Consensus of opinion, however, is that paludrine is still the drug of choice and in case of strains like the African mentioned above paludrine monohydrochloride should be reinforced with mepacrine or chloroquine. It may be added that the action of paludrine is less rapid than quinine, mepacrine and chloroquine, especially in *P. vivax* infection. In emergencies therefore its use alone is unsuitable. M-594 (N_1-*l*:4 dichlorophenyl-N^3-isopropyl diguanide) is reported to be more active than paludrine and clinical trails are in progress.

Sulphonamides

Sulphonamides have been referred to as effective in *P. knowlesi* in Rhesus monkey (Coggshell 1938), and S. diazine, S. merazine, and S. thiazole as suppressive in *P. gallinaceum* infection in fowls. S. diazine, S. merazine and S. metazine are stated to be most promising in human malaria, especially in *P. falsiparum* (Covell 1943).

Drugs fouud with no effect on malaria

Investigations done at the Malaria Institute of India showed that the following drugs have no effect on malaria :

Alstonia scholaris, A-Gad, Antique, Quine Chirvasal, Coffee Husk, Degan's remedy, Fraxine malacophylla, Hindscout, HT7, Jwaraghna, Saptaparna, Karanjiwa seeds, Lichtenstcin cure, malaridol, Sunine, Tinospora cordifolia, Vitex peduncularis.

Drugs of Choice

It will be seen from the above that quinine, mepacrine, chloroquine and allied 4-aminoquinolines, and proguanil are effective in the treatment of the clinical attacks of malaria. Chloroquine and proguanil are at present the drugs of choice. In relapsing vivax malaria concurrent treatment with quinine and 8-aminoquinoline such as isopentaquine, may be preferable.

Suppressive Treatment

It is generally agreed that the following drugs will effectively suppress malaria :

Drug	Dose	Remarks
Mepacrine hydrochloride	*Non-immune* 0.1 g. daily (preferably with build up of 0.3 g. daily for 5 days)	The daily dose to be continued in case of falsiparum for at least three weeks after exposure.
	Partially immune 0.2 g. twice weekly or 0.3 g. weekly may be useful for mass prophylaxis where the intensity of malaria is not very high. 0.1 g. daily is most satisfactory.	
Chloroquine disphosphate	0.3 to .25 g. base once weekly on the same day of the week.	
Proguanil	0.3 g. once a week in hyperendemic areas. In other areas 0.1 g. to 0.3 g. weekly have given promising results.	

Quinine is the least effective as a suppressive drug. Chloroquine and proguanil offer the best margins of safety.

The suppressive treatment should be given with discretion after carefully considering all relevant factors. In emergencies as when a large group of labourers or troops have to operate in malarious areas the suppressive treatment is obviously indicated. Before suppressive treatment is discontinued one must make sure that facilities for treatment and hospitalisation are available and that the work in hand will not suffer if a large number of men go down with malaria.*

*" The problem of chloroquine resistance of *P. falsiparum*, observed first in Assam in 1973 and later in some other parts of the country and trials with different drugs led to changes in recommended treatment of malaria cases. The drug policy of the National Malaria Programme, as given below, is proposed to be continued for the present, with emphasis on "the immediate treatment of malarial cases by multipurpose workers" and community participation will be ensured by extending these drug Distribution Centres and Fever Treatment Depots network in rural areas".

Presumptive Treatment in Chloroquine Resistance *P. falciparum* Cases (All fever Cases current or with history) :

Active Case Detection Passive Case Detection	Amodiaquine 600 mg base (adult) Sulphalene 1000 mg dose and Pyrimethamine 50 mg dose.
Drug Distribution Centres and Fever Treatment Depots	Amodiaquine 600 mg. base (adult)

Note : Full dose is to be given at a time after meals. Children 0-1, 2-4, 5-8, 9-14 will recieve 1/8, 1/4, 1/2 and 3/4 of the adult dose respectively.

Radical Treatment (*P. falciparum*, Chloroquine Resistant Areas):

Sulphalene 1000 mg dose and Pyrimethamine 50 mg dose, along with Primaquine 45 mg base for adult. The children except infants will recieve the drug in proportionately small doses. Infants and pregnant women need not be given any Primaquine.
(Sulphalene dose is given in two tablets).

(Radical treatment for *P. vivax*. *P. malariae* or mixed *P. vivax* and *P. malariae* : Chloroquine 600 mg base on the first day and Primaquine 15 mg base daily for five days).

Areas where P. falsiparum is sensitive to Chloroquine

(*i*) Presumptive treatment by Active Case Detection ; Passive Case Detection Chloroquino 600 mg base for adults. Drug Distribution Centres Fever Treatment Depots.

(*Footnote contd. to next page*)

(*Footnote contd. from previous page*)

(*ii*) Adult	Chloroquine 600 mg+Primaquine 45 mg (Single dose)

Radical Treatment of *P. Vivax/P. Malariae* or Mixed

1st Day : Chloroquine 600 mg+Primaquine 15 mg.
2nd day-5th day : Primaquine 15 mg only daily.

Drug schedule for labour population in *P. falciparum* Containment Programme PfCP Areas

Labourer before leaving

PfCP Area (Zone 1 or any area with high incidence of Pf	Chloroquine 600 mg+Primaquine 45 mg (adult single dose) Mass Administration
Labourer coming from Zone I and on Detection in Zone II and III	Presumptive : Chloroqnine 600 mg+Primaquine 45 mg Radical : Chloroquine 1500 mg in three divided doses and Primaquine 45 mg adult single dose on first day. If no respone to this regime within three days (72 hours) Sulphalene 1000 mg Pyrimethamine 50 mg with Primaquine 45 mg. Primaquine will not be given to infants and Pregnant women.

General

Drug Distribution Centres will not distribute Paracetamol.

Active Case Distribution/Passive Case Detection ? Fever Treatment Depots will give Paracetamol 600 mg (adult) for use only in fever cases. Sulphate/Hydrochloride Preparation of quinine salts are life saving in cases where other drugs fail. For actual cerebral or other serious types of malaria intravenous preparations should be used.

Chloroquine injectables : Special precautions should be taken for the use of this in children, as shock may be produced. In

Chloroquine resistant areas *P. falciparum* cases should not be treated with Chloroquine"

(*Footnote contd. to next page*)

(*Footnote contd. from previous page*)

(*Source* : Narasimham, M.V.V.L., *National Malaria Eradication Programme*, National Health Programme Series 4, Gupta, J.P. and Bhatnagar, S. Series Editors, National Institute of Health and Family Welfare, New Delhi, 1988).

REFERENCES

Acton, H. W., (1920) *Trop. Dis. Bull.* 16, 328.

Acton, H. W., Cwajel, D. F., and Dewey, J.O. (1921) *Ind. J. Med. Res.*, 8, 861-867.

Acton, H. W., and Knowles, R. (1924) *Ind. Med. Gaz.*, 59, 177-184.

Berkely Hill O. A. R. (1926), *Ibid.*, 61, 231-232.

Black, R. H. (1949), *R. Tr. Soc. Trop. Med. Hyg.* 42, 565-68.

Ciuca, M., Irimesee, G., Munoliu, E., Alexa and Constantinese (1926) *Trop. Dis. Bull.* 23, 546.

Cordes (1924) *Ibid.*. 21, 856.

Covell, G., (1943) *J. Mal. Inst. Ind.* 5, 135.

Idem (1949) *Brit. Med. J.*, Oct. 8, 2, 773.

Field, J. W. (1938) *Bull. Inst. Med. Res.* F. M. S., 2, 21.

Federated Malaya States Government Press 1939.

Fletcher, W. (1925) *Trop. Dis. Bull.* 23, 545.

Hicks, E.P., and Dewan Chand (1935) Rec. *Mal. Surv. Ind.* 5, 39-50.

James, S. P. (1927) *Brit. Med. J.* Aug. 27, 340-343.

Joglekar, G. V. (1940) *Ind. Med. J.* 39, 291-296, 35, 25-26.

Mac Gilchrist (1915) *Ind. J. Med. Res.* 3, 1-89.

Moulder, J. W. (1950) *Trop. Dis. Bull.* 47, 118.

Napier, L. E. (1946) *Ibid.*, 43, 10-11.

Notes of *Malaria Conference held at the Malaria Institute of India*, November 1949.

Prain, D. (1924) *Brit. Med. J.* 1023-1024.

Pranger, P., and Filer M. K. (1948) *Ann. Inst. Pasteur.* 75, 329-337.

Privy Council Special Report Series 96, Med. Res. Council, 1925.

Seabra, P. (1950) *Trop. Dis. Bull.* 47, 438.

Taliaferro, W. H. (1949) *Ibid.*, 46, 1122.

For work on Paludrine refer to the paper on "Researches on Paludrine in Malaria" by Professor Fairly discussed in the Royal Society of Tropical Medicine and Hygiene on June 20, 1946 ; See also *Lancet*. November 1946, p. 640.

10

Progress Made

Ross made the epoch-making discovery of the mosquito malaria theory over 50 years ago.* He was bitterly disappointed to see that no use was subsequently being made of his findings, even in the land where the discovery was made. He poured out his bitterness on page 77 of his poem "The anniversary 1917". Watson in his Finlayson memorial lecture explained the "lag period" in the following words : "Viewed in the light of the year 1934 we must regret what happened nearly 40 years ago......the explanation is simple that the idea of public health grew slowly in the minds of Governments—both the Indian and British Governments were slow to realise what might be achieved". In the last one decade or two great interest has been taken in the malaria problem. War in the East gave further impetus to the study of malaria. Anti-malaria work done in Klang, Swettenham, the great swamps of Malaya, Carey Islands, Singapore, Panama and other places attracted the attention of all those interested in public health problems. The achievements of William Crawford Gorgas in the early twentieth century in Panama, in the words of Sir Malcolm Watson, were "the greatest sanitary achievement the world has seen". The Rocke-

*20 August 1897 in Secunderabad.

feller Foundation concentrated its attention upon solving the malaria problem over 25 years ago and opened a school for teaching and research of malaria at Leisberg in Georgia in 1922 with Darling as Director and Barber as his associate. "He brought in more precise and effective methods for controlling malaria, and inspired a note of usefulness, especially drawing attention to 'species control', and standardised the measuring of the amount of malaria by taking spleen rates". Darlings association with the League of Nations gave an entirely new orientation to the antimalaria campaign throughout the world. The quinine therapy for malaria control was given up and anti-mosquio control took its place. The Rockefeller Foundation further granted scholarships to medical men from many countries to go round different parts of the world where antimalaria work was being carried out. In 1923, at the request of the Italian Government, the Foundation sent Hackett to Italy, to do a general survey of malaria, assisted by Misseroli. The work at Port Torres in Sardinia proved a great success (1925), and a few year later, Mussolini started his famous work of reclaiming the Bontine marshes. Researches made and experience gained by various workers in different parts of the world considerably affected the work in India. In 1927, at a Congress of the Far Eastern Association of Tropical Medicine, held at Calcutta, Watson laid great stress on anti-malaria measures.

Killing of adult mosquitoes with pyrethrum, the discovery of DDT and recent introduction of drugs like paludrine, chloroquine followed in quick succession. The Malaria Institute of India, Ross Institute of Tropical Hygiene, India Branch, various antimalaria organisations in States and numerous field units have done splendid work. In addition to carrying out researches in malaria control and the study of allied subject, the Malaria Institute of India during 1940-45 trained 630 medical officers both Civil and Defence Service Officers and Antimalaria Assistants, 426 members of the Indian Hospital Corps and Sanitary Inspectors. In addition 87 Engineers also got special training during this period.

In 1943 the Government of India appointed a Health Survey and Development Committee to make a broad survey of the recent position in regard to health conditions and health organization and to make recommendations for the future. The Committee recommended amongst other things (*i*) establishment of malaria control organisation at the headquarters of each province with a number of malaria control units each under a medical officer, especially trained in antimalaria work, for operating in the affected areas in different parts of the provinces, (*ii*) provision of trained staff in adequate number, (*iii*) supply of drugs, appliances and other requirements for carrying out antimalaria campaigns effectively, (*iv*) production of antimalaria drugs without delay, raising of quinine production to the pre-war level of consumption in India from indigenous bark, (*v*) production of mepacrine in India for 30 million patients, (*vi*) expansion of pyrethrum production, (*vii*) strengthening of the staff of the Malaria Institute of India to enable it to fulfil its important task of advising provincial administrations in the development of antimalaria measures, of co-ordinating such work in the provinces and of training the higher types of malaria personnel, and (*viii*) equitable basis of distribution of antimalaria drugs on reasonable cost, so that they are available to the poorest class all over the country.

It is very encouraging to find that the recommendations* have not only been accepted in principle but that malaria control has been given priority by the Government of India. The World Health Organisation is also aiming to mobilise all the resources for "the eradication of malaria from the world".

*In April 1953, the National Malaria Control Programme was launched. The major focus was on "intensive residual insecticide spray" in malarious areas of the country. Bilateral and multilateral agencies provided assistance. The Malaria Institute of India was designated as coordinating agency for all authorities and their activities.

The Malaria Institute of India was a unique institution. In 1909 the Malaria Bureau was established financed by the Indian Research

(*Footnote contd. to next page*)

(Footnote contd. from previous page)

Fund Association. In 1927, it was developed as a central organisation and named as Malaria Survey of India. In 1938 the name of the organisation was changed to the Malaria Institute of ndia. In 1940 it was taken over by the Government of India. Colonel Sir S. Richard Christophers, C. I. E., F. R. S., I. M. S. concieved the idea of a broad based central malaria organisation. It was further developed by a series of distinguished officers of the Indian Medical Service, and a number of scientists on the staff of the institute in the early stages, notably by Lieut. Colonel J. A. Sinton, V. C., O. B. E. I. M. S. and Major-General Sir Gordon Covell, C. I. E., I. M. S.

In 1940, Government of India took over the Institute. The Indian Reseach Fund Association continued to finance research activities, till 1946. Dr. M.C. Balfour, Regional Director in the Far East International Health Division of the Rockfeller Foundation at the Fourth International Congress on Tropical Medicine and Malaria in 1948, called it "as the driving force in studies of malariology and in the promotion of malaria control in the Far East". (For further details see on Activities of the Malaria Institute of India during World War II by Lieut.-Colonel Jaswant Singh and in Raina, B. L. ed. *Preventive Medicine* (Nutrition, Malaria Control and Prevention of Diseases) Official History of The Indian Armed Forces in the Second World War 1939-45. Medical Services, Combined Inter-Services Historical Section India & Pakistan. 1961).

The results of the National Malaria Control Programme were very encouraging. In April 1958, the malaria programme was further developed. The residual spraying was extended throughout the country. The extended programme was called National Malaria Eradication Programme. It had three phases, *viz.* attack, consolidation and maintenance. (No preparatory phase was needed as the National Malaria Control Phase was virtuality the Preparatory Phase). Its notable features included : intensive, extensive and closely superv sed residual spraying ; surveillance operations (from the third year), visiting houses twice a month specifically for surviellance) for early detection of malaria cases and their treatment and tracing the origin of infection, till malaria is eradicated ; gradual discontinuation of residual spraying as control is achieved : transfering the responsbility for maintenance to States as a part of normal health system ; coordination of malaria control activities with neighbouring countries ; assistance of international agencies bilateral and multilateral like UNICEF, WHO, USTCMP, Rockfeller Foundation, SIDA ; development of a nationwide malaria eradication organisation with augmented staff at all levels in the States

(Footnote contd. to next page)

(Footnote contd. from previous page)

(separate staff for spraying and surviellance) regional coordinating organisation at Baroda, Conoor, Cuttak, Delhi, Hyderabad, Shillong and a separate Directorate at the Centre. The role of Malaria Institute of India changed in 1958 and was limited mainly to research, training, and dissemination of technical information.

Early in 1960s reports started accumulating that the malarial parasite in humans disappears after about three years continued protection. Alarming repots also started coming of mosquitoes acquiring resistance to insecticides. From 1965, the malaria incidence started increasing. In addition to resistence of varying degrees to insecticides by some vectors, areas with *P. falciparum* resistant to chloroquine were reported. Besides the resistence of vectors to insecticides and parasite to chloroquine, the set-back to malaria programme was due to a number of other reasons such as unpreparedness of the State Government to assume responsibility for malaria control during maintenance phase mainly because of weaknesses in the health infrastructure, financial constraints, logistics and managerial problems, unpreparedness of malaria programme personnel for their new roles and such other factors.

The incresse in the incidence of malaria cases led to emergence of Modified Plan of Operation in 1976, which included among other activities, *P. falciparum* containment programme. By this time, like in other health and family welfare programmes, the need for greater real people's participation, health education, multisectorial coordination, and comprehensive primary health care was realised. There was also greater appreciation of bio-environmental approach to malaria control. Chemotherapeutic measures and programmes as already mentioned. were developed based on experience and research.

The measures that are being undertaken in May 1990 ' for control of malaria through vector control are : (*i*) application of chemicals such as mosquito larvicidal oil/fenthion/Paris green/tenephos in water collections to eliminate the aquatic stages of mosquitoes ; (*ii*) space spraying of 0.1 per cent pyrethrum extract in and around 50 houses of every malaria case to kill infected vectors (mosquitoes responsible for transmission of malaria) and reduction of breeding sources through minor engineering methods and bio-environmental control methods such as introduction of mosquito larvae eating fish in breeding places wherever feasible". (Written Reply by Minister of State for Health and Family Welfare Shri Rasheed Masood to a question by Professor K. V. Thomas, in the Lok Sabha on 23 May 1990. PIB).

Postscript

The happiness and prosperity of the people are closely connected with the degree of the health which they enjoy. Varied aspects of public health problems are intimately, related to the social and economic conditions of the people, the availability of trained personnel, material and equipment, the extent of the country's capacity, a co-ordinative machinery and adequate control to ensure carrying out of plans, experiments and research.

India, despite its rich natural resources, is a very poor country, poor in goods, poor in education, poor in health. The per capita income in 1939-40 was Rs. 67/- per year. During 1946-47 it was Rs. 228/-,* On such a low income people have to eat, clothe themselves and live. In pre-war days the cost of the cheapest balanced diet alone was Rs. 48/- to Rs. 72/- per head per year. The cost of living has considerably increased since.** Education is poor, about 88 per cent of the

*Per Capita Net National Product (Rupees) in India at current, prices increased from 245.5 (1950-51) to 3284 (1987-88). The percentage of population below the poverty line in India estimated for 1983-84 is 37.4.

**Index number of wholesale prices in March 1950 was approximately as follows :

(Base year ending August 1939 = 100)

General index	...	...	392.4
Food articles	...	...	396.2
Cereals	...	...	454.0
Cereals	...	...	440.0

people being illiterate. Health education is poorer still. Doctors and nurses are limited. Only about one doctor to 6000 and one nurse to 43,000 are available.* Facilities for specialist training and research are patchy. Coupled with such an unfortunate economic and educational background, the standard, of public health is one of the lowest in the world. Famines and epidemics are not infrequent. The following figures for 1937** quoted by Grant (1944) tell a tragic story :

	Expectation of life	Death rate per 1000 population	Infant mortality per 1000 births
Australia	67 years	9.4	38
England & Wales	63 ,,	12.4	58
Japan	47 ,,	17.0	106
Undivided India	27 ,,	22.4	162

The rises in prices has been continuing. In India the wholesale price index (base 1981-82=100) in the week ending September 15, 1990 reported was 180.2. The index for primary articles including food was 184.8 (PTI).

The picture of sickness due to malaria has changed since 1951. It is difficult to draw morbidity picture in India, for a number of reasons. The morbidity picture of insured persons under the Employees State Insurance Scheme may present a trend of prevalence of diseases in this group of population.

During 1986-87 the number of New cases per 1000 insured persons of the gastro-intestinal and respiratory disorders were higher than malaria : Malaria cases were 23.2, as against 262.8 dysentry all forms, common cold 227, bronchitis 204.8, diarrhoe and enteritis 141.4, diseases of stomach and duodenum 123.5 other diseases of digestive system 107.3.

Source : ESI Corporation, cited in Health Information India, 1988. Malaria Positive Cases in India in 1987 were 1,663,284.

*1980s situation. (*see Footnote next page*)

**1990 situation. (*see Footnote next page*)

In India, (1951) amongst the preventable diseases, malaria claims first place importance. It is doubly unfortunate that to a great extent malaria is the creation of man.

(*Footnote contd. from previous page*)

***Population per physician and midwife/nurse in Bangladesh, India and Pakistan in 1980s.**

Country	Population per Physician		Population per Midwife Nurse	
	Year	Number	Year	Number
Bangladesh	1981	8,908	1981	15,005
India	1985	2,649	1985	2,038
Pakistan	1981	3,172	1981	4,492

Source : "WHO" in *Pocket Book on Family Welfare Information.* Department of Family Wefare. Ministry of Health and Family Welfare. Government of India, New Delhi, 1988.

****Life Expectancy at Birth (years); Birth Rate Per 1000 population ; and Infant Mortality Per 1000 live Births for Australia, United Kingdom, Japan, Bangladesh, India and Pakistan**

Country	Life Expectancy Male	Female	Death Rate	Infant Mortality
Australia	**72**	**78.2**	**7.6**	**9.8**
United Kingdom	**71,9**	**77.6**	**12.4**	**9.4**
Japan	**75.5**	**81.6**	**6.5**	**5.2**
Bangladesh	**47.5**	**47**	**17.5**	**104,7**
Pakisthan	**53.4**	**51.7**	**15.3**	**119.8**
India	**54,1**	**54.7**	**12.3**	**95**

Source : *World Health Statistics—1987* W.H.O. cited in *Health Information India 1988.* C.B.H.I. Dte G.H.S. Ministry of Health & F.W., New Delhi.

The responsibility for public health administration lies mostly on Provincial, now State Governments. But the control of the Stated Governments over local bodies is so weak that not much progress has been made. The report of the Simon Commission (1930) is worth repetition, "The result of the legislative and administrative action taken in accordance with the scheme of the reforms was in effect to deprive the new Ministers of local self-governments of powers which were essential if they were to perform their task successfully".

As to the urban population, the report of the second meeting of the Central Advisory Board of Health 1939 recorded that "According to available information, nearly half the districts and three quarters of the municipalities in British India are still without qualified health officers. In many of the areas visited by us we have been unfavourably impressed with the standard of health administration and with the manner in which these duties have been performed. Health Officers are to be found in most of the larger municipalities, but their work is too often ineffective because they have incomplete control of the health organisation, or because their recommendations fail to recieve active consideration from their councils". A few municipalities and corporations like Bombay are notable exceptions. It is obvious that scientific, preventive and curative services are still beyond the reach of 80 per cent of the men, women and childern of India. Progress has been made in the last few years but it has been patchy and limited to isolated areas. Taking India as a whole the menace of malaria is no less than it was before, as is evident from all-India mortality and morbidity figures.* With the brief account set out in previous sections in mind, one is forced to the conclusion that the malaria problem cannot be adequately solved without the solution of economic, educational and other vital problems referred to above. The message of health can be brought home to the people not by preaching alone, but also by provi-

*Mortality and morbidity picture has changed as indicated earlier but malaria has not yet lost to "sting".

ding facilities to put into practice what they are taught. It is futile to ask a poor farmer to use mosquito nets or canvas mosquito boots, so long as he cannot afford more than a loin-cloth and a pair of old sandals (*chappals*)—the latter usually to be kept tied at the end of the stick resting on his shoulder to prevent wear and tear and used only when absolutely necessary while walking on hot sand or thorny ground. A malariologist obviously cannot plough his solitary furrow. He has to take the help of the economist, the educationist, the agriculturist, the engineer, the lawyer and the State. Consideration of vast and varied problems is essential for the study of the health problem of a country in its true perspective. It must be emphasised that large tracts of land can be brought under cultivation if malaria problem is solved.

The solution of the malaria problem in India requires the serious consideration of five principal factors, *viz*., (1) education, (2) organisation, (3) medical protection, (4) legislation, and (5) funds.

(1) Education

(*a*) Health education must form a part of general education and should be appropriate for the age of the child.

(*b*) The sanitary conscience of the public should be awakened by intensive and extensive propaganda. Propaganda by means of leaflets, pamphlets, posters, exhibition, films, etc. has its own utility. but unaided by practical demonstration, it hardly serves its purpose, as most of the people do not comprehend what exactly the leaflet contains or the poster denotes. For propaganda to become successful, practical demonstrations are essential Medical men can form an all-India Anti-malaria Association. Such an Association can play a very effective role.

(*c*) Malaria should be introduced as a special subject in all the medical schools and colleges of India. A chair for teaching malariology should be introduced in the universities. Even if only one question on malaria is asked in an examination paper of Hygiene and Public Health, it will stimulate the interest of medical students in malariology. Facilities for field work and research work should be available for the post-graduates in all universities. Refresher courses for already qualified medical personnel will prove of great value. A large number of medical men, engineers, malaria assistants and inspectors will be required. Every registered medical practitioner can be kept informed on current ideas concerning malaria control through circulars by a Central Health Organization.

(2) Organization

Malaria control should be centralised and not left entirely to the local bodies. A scheme more or less on the following lines can ensure efficiency and uniformity.

(*a*) *Central Board of Malaria Control.* The members of the Board can be selected by the Central Advisory Board of Health and should include amongst others a Consultant in malariology. There should be a Director of Malaria Control in India, who can work as Secretary to the Central Board, and through him the Board can exercise executive control over the States. The Board can draw out a 15-year plan in collaboration with the World Health Organisation for dealing with the menace of malaria, and should ensure that it is carried out.

(*b*) State Governments should have a Deputy Director of Malaria, who will be directly responsible through the Director of Public Health to the Director of Malaria Control, India. The State Governments should have a State Malaria Control Board, which should include the Minister of Public Health, the Director of Public Health, the Chief Engineer, Directors of Agriculture, Fisheries, Botanical Gardens, the Finance Minister and Conservator of Forests. Representatives of Zamindars, Industries, Railways and Municipalities can be co-opted. The Deputy Director, Malaria Control, can act as Secretary.

(*c*) Districts or a group of districts should have an Assistant Director, Malaria Control, with a mobile field laboratory consisting among others, an entomologist. When the preliminary surveys are completed, the field laboratories may be kept only in one or two districts in the State (except those which are non-malarious). Every district should have an antimalaria committee, more or less on the same lines as State Committees. A detailed health survey, including an entomological survey, of the whole of the inhabited parts of India is essential. This should be started in hyperendemic malarious areas first. All constructions of roads, canals, factories and residential buildings ought to be approved by a malariologist.

(*d*) In every sub division endemic or hyperendemic districts or in Tehsils there should be an antimalaria officer and an antimalaria committee. Staff for malaria control will obviously not be necessary in malaria free areas. It may be stated that some States have already started Malaria Control Organisations.

(3) Medical Protection

For the treatment of 100 to 200 million sufferers from malaria, qualified medical men, hospital accommodation, nursing facilities and necessary quantities of quinine and synthetic drugs are required. It was estimated that there were only 47,500 doctors and 7,000 nurses in United India and if one doctor for 2,000 of population is necessary, India will require 185,000 doctors. Adequate planning for the production of drugs like quinine and proguanil is essential. It is estimated that the quantity of quinine required for India is about 1.5 million pounds. The quantity consumed in pre-war years was about 210,000 pounds, out of which only about 70,000 pounds was manufactured in India. Parts of Assam, Bengal, Orissa, Bhutan, Sikkim, Madras, Travancore, Cochin, Mysore and

Coorg are suitable for cinchona cultivation. It is reported that 38,000 acres of land (each acre capable of producing 100 to 200 pounds of quinine per year) are available in India. It will be observed from the above figures that India can not only become self-supporting for its quinine, but can produce ten times its requirements (Krishnan 1940). The recently discovered chemotherapeutic agents have now, to a great extent, replaced quinine. Their manufacture in the country will require change in cinchona cultivation policy. There is no reason why chemical and pharmaceutical industry should not be able to produce drugs for India's need. In view of their therapeutic value we must now work out carefully our requirement for malaria control (stores, equipment and drugs) and plan their production in the country. Production of quinine may be necessary for the time being till the country starts producing the new chemotherapeutic agents in sufficient quantity to meet the total requirement. Their distribution will require considerable planning, and can be done by the Central Malaria Control Board. Apart from curative drugs, large quantities of DDT, suitable mixtures of oils, paris green and pyrethrum, etc , will be required for malaria control. Pyrethrum requires a high altitude with a dry climate and well drained soil, and it is very encouraging to find that it can be successfully cultivated in Kulu, Palampur, Kashmir and Nilgiris. It is estimated that 15,000 short tons (2000 lbs. for a ton) will be required for India's need per year. This will require 120,000 acres of land to produce. Once DDT and other new insecticides in sufficient quantity become available in the country the cultivation of pyrethrum can be reduced or completely replaced by other crops. Economic aspect of malaria control measures is vital. With the assistance of the World Health Organisation supplies can be arranged for the time being from abroad at reasonable cost.

(4) Legislation

Discussing public health services, the Supreme Court Justice, John M. Harlan, observed that "it is the settled doctrine of this court that as a Government is organised for the purpose among others of preserving the public health, and public morals, it cannot divest itself of the responsibility of providing these objects". Consolidated laws must be enacted and enforced to ensure that health rules laid down by the experts are carried out.

(5) **Funds**

Local bodies have neither the resources nor the money to finance malaria control scheme on a large scale. They may be able to meet only a small portion of the expenses ; the rest will have to be shared between the States and the Central Government. The Central Malaria Control Organisation should be allotted necessary funds, and should have the powers to allot money to the States, according to their respective requirements. There is no doubt that in the beginning expenses will be high, but every rupee spent will mean thousands of rupees saved, together with the preservation of thousands of lives, and the prevention of the untold miseries endured by malaria sufferers. No price is too great for ensuring public health security. The interdepartmental committee, to co-ordinate health and welfare activities (a co-ordination which is an essential part of any health programme) in the U.S.A. observed in their report for 1939. "It is the conviction of the Committee, derived from experience, that at the present time there is no greater public need from the standpoint of individual and social security than a comprehensive programme to safeguard a nation's health". It is an observation which is true for any part of the world.*

*"The centralization and decentralization" of health programmes, and disease specific vertical approach and comprehensive health approach have been subjects of debate now for some years. The medical history supports both approaches. There was criticism of launching a separate anti-malaria programme in the Second World War. The experience showed that the selective programme reduced mortality and morbidity due to malaria and contributed to victory of the Allied Forces in the Eastern Theatre of war. There may be occasions when urgency to control a disease or disorder of menacing proportions demands launching a disease specific vertical programme, as demonstrated from the impact of such a

(*Footnote contd. to next page*)

REFERENCES

Grant, J. B., (1944) *Health of India*, Oxford University Press, Bombay.

Krishnan, K. V., (1940) *Bengal Public Health Journal*, 2, 1.

(*Footnote contd. from previous page*)

programme in the World War II. Further experience of health and family planning programmes also beckons that if and when such an approach is adopted it should not only be for a limited period, but also be so designed that it can smoothly become part of the comprehensive health care system and the comprehensive health care system should have the strength to undertake the additional responsibilities. In the normal circumstances, we have to agree with Debabar Banerjee that "The Primary health care is based on the people, rather than pre-determined system. It emphasises social control over health services, involving people at all stages of health service development, namely problem identification, programme formation, programme implementation and evaluation. Selective primary health care is thus a contradiction in terms, because it adopts an authoritarian or paternalistic approach in selecting for others a number of limited vertical health programmes and leaves the other causes of illhealth untouched". ("Primary Health Care Selective or Comprehensive Approach" in *World Health Forum*. 5(4) World Health Organisation Geneva, 1984). It may be added that the expression "involving people" is not as simple as it sounds. It involves : (*i*) combating basic human weakness to resist sharing power ; (*ii*) creating "opportunities that enable all members of the community and the larger society to actively contribute to and influence the development process and share equitably in the fruits of development"; (*iii*) helping to upgrade the knowledge and skills of the community leaders in discovering the important aspects of the problems, planning programmes to solve, implement, monitor and evaluate them ; (*iv*) providing financial and other resources and professional support required by the community ; and (*v*) building checks and balances to prevent groups with vested interests taking special advantage and eroding the principles of equity.

Appendices

APPENDIX A

EXTRACTS FROM THE REPORT OF HEALTH SURVEY AND DEVELOPMENT COMMITTEE

In recent years even more effective preventive measures against malaria have become available, including potent chemicals for the destruction of the mosquito and drugs for protecting man against repeated infection. The remarkable manner in which the fighting forces of the Allies operating in highly malarious tracts have been protected against this scourge during the present war again bears testimony to the possibility of effectively controlling the disease. It is clear to us that, given the determination, the money and the requisite staff, it should be possible to reduce the incidence of the disease in India to small proportions.

ANTIMALARIA MEASURES

The measures that are necessary against malaria fall under two main heads, namely : (1) those which are directed against the transmitter of infection, the mosquito, and (2) those which deal with man in his two-fold capacity as a victim of the disease and as a reservoir of infection. Antimosquito measures may be grouped under the following heads :

(*i*) those which control the breeding of the mosquito ; and

(*ii*) those which are directed against the insect in its adult form.

Measures to control the breeding of mosquitoes. These measures take a wide variety of forms, although the main principles involved are the same, *viz.*, the obliteration of facilities for the laying of eggs by the female mosquito and the creation of conditions inimical to the survival of the insect in its larval stage in circumstances when egg-laying cannot be prevented. The steps that are necessary for these purposes include, among others, drainage to prevent accumulations of water canalisation of water channels and the removal of vegetation from their sides, the use of larvicides such as mineral oils, paris green and the more recent synthetic product D.D.T., selective clearing of jungle or shading of water courses in certain cases aed the use of larvivorous fish.

There are many varieties of fish in this country which prey on mosquito larvae. Gambusia, an American species of minnow, introduced into India about twenty years ago, is being used in the wells in Bangalore and Bombay, the ornamental waters in Delhi and in many other parts of the country. This species has been proved to possess all the qualities required for antimosquito work and is probably more suitable for this purpose than any other species. It should be emphasised, however, that the value of fish is very limited. They are useful in artificial collections of water like ornamental waters but their use is of doubtful value as a general antilarval measure.

For dealing with the malarial conditions created by large constructional works and irrigation projects, well-planned schemes requiring considerable technical supervision and heavy expenditure will be necessary These can obviously be undertaken and carried out only by the State. On the other hand, in many parts of the rural areas, effective results may be secured by works of a minor nature, such as the filling up of pools and ditches so as to prevent collections of water or other measures already mentioned such as oiling, removal of vegetation, etc. In our short-term programme, we have made certain suggestions for the carrying out of such measures in rural areas. We have provided for a small labour force of 15 in each primary unit one of whose duties will be to see to the carrying out of these minor works. These men may be unable to deal effectively with the whole area covered by such a unit, but an important part of their work will lie in their being able, as a trained group, to demonstrate to the villagers how to go about these tasks properly. We hope that the village Committees we have recommended will be able to mobilise voluntary local effort in carrying out such measures and that we shall thus be able to enlist a tremendous force in the fight against this disease. The small labour squad will also form the nucleus round which, during an epidemic, an expanded organisation can be rapidly built up.

It is desirable that the planning and execution of these antimalarial works should, as far as possible, receive technical guidance and we have recommended the appointment of an Assistant Public Health Engineer at the headquarters of each secondary unit for this purpose. Direct local supervision will be provided by the medical officer in charge of the primary unit and his two public health inspectors.

Although we hope that the local effort we have referred to will help to reduce the cost of labour, sufficient public funds should be made available to ensure that the required expenditure will be fully met. We have included in our budget for each primary unit a provision for meeting this expenditure.

Measures against the adult mosquito. The Director, Malaria Institute of India, has pointed out that the results of spray-killing operations carried out in various parts of the country hold out the hope that "we have at last a weapon which, when its full possibilities have been developed, will prove effective for rural. as well as urban and industrial, malaria". Pyrethrin, the active principle extracted from the flower of the pyrethrum plant, has been found to be an effective insecticide and has been used extensively as a spray for the killing of adult mosquitoes. The synthetic product, D.D.T., has provided an even effective insecticide than pyrethrum. The great advantage of D.D.T. over pyrethrum is its residual effect, while pyrethrum is superior to D.D.T. in its immediate knock-down effect. A combination of the two products has been tried on a relatively small scale and found to give satisfactory results. The purpose of this measure is to kill infected mosquitoes and to reduce the longivity of mosquitoes in an area, so that the number which live long enough to become malaria carriers is reduced to the minimum. This measure has been developed during the last few years and is of special value where antilarval measures may take too long to give results, or as a supplement to such measures.

These operations against the adult mosquito will be undertaken in the rural areas by the squads of 15 labourers that have been provided in each primary unit with, we hope, the active support and assistance of the villagers.

We shall deal with the subject of ensuring adequate supplies of these insecticides for the the use of the health departments in India later in this chapter.

MEASURES IN RELATION TO MAN

(*a*) Man as a Victim of the Disease

Treatment. Here the primary need is to ensure adequate treatment. This involves a proper diagnosis where possible and a sufficient supply of the requisite drugs. While it may not be practicable to have a microscope at every primary health centre, it should be possible to send blood-smears for examination, when necessary, to the nearest 30 bed hospital and obtain a diagnosis without undue delay. During times of epidemics, however, the primary need will be for the immediate distribution of antimalarial drugs.

Quinine has for long been the drug of choice in the treatment of malaria. More recently, atebrin (or mepacrine as it is now being called) has also come widely into use. After an extended study of the comparative values of quinine and atebrin for the treatment of the disease, the Malaria Commission of the League of Nations came to the conclusion in their fourth report (1937) that, while atebrin was more effective against certain species of the parasite, quinine was more potent against others. In India, under the conditions arising out of the War, many millions of tablets of mepacrine have been widely distributed among the general population for the mass treatment of malaria in view of a shortage in the supply of quinine. So far no untoward results have been definitely substantiated from this widespread use of the drug, though careful investigation in regard to the matter will no doubt have to be continued. Further, experience of the distribution of this drug to Allied fighting forces in the Tropics under conditions, which preclude any degree of control over its use by the individual, has also led to the conclusion that it can be used with safety for mass treatment. Recent investigations suggest that an even more effective synthetic product, paludrine, is likely to come into use at an early date. In these circumstances, there is the possibility that synthetic products may, in due course, come to replace, to an appreciable extent, the use of quinine as the routine drug for the treatment of malaria.

Other measures. The use of quinine and mepacrine as suppressive agents for preventing the development of malaria has been extensively tried among troops continuously exposed to infection in highly malarious areas. The consensus of opinion appears to be that quinine has but small value as a suppressive agent, the reason probably being that it is excreted quickly and does not, therefore, remain in sufficient concentration in the circulation. Mepacrine has, on the other hand, a much slower rate of excretion and has been found to be more effective than quinine when used for this purpose.

The question of production of adequate quantities of quinine and of mepacrine for the needs of the country will be discussed later.

Equally important is the question of affording protection to a healthy person against the bite of an infected mosquito. The measures that are generally adopted include, in addition to the killing of the adult mosquitoes, the use of mosquito repellents on exposed parts of the body and of mosquito nets and mosquito coils with pyrethrum as the base as well as the screening of houses so as to prevent the entry of the insect. These are all undoubtedly useful but, as measures for the general population in malarious places, they seem to be of limited practical application.

(*b*) Man as a Reservoir of Infection

The life of the parasite is passed partly in man and partly in the mosquito. In man it exists in two forms, namely, one which undergoes the asexual type of reproduction during which the malarial attack is produced and the other, the male and female sexual elements, which on ingestion by the mosquito, unite and by further development in that insect, give it the power of infecting man. Plasmoquine has been found to be effective in killing these sexual forms when they circulate in man's blood. In these circumstances, a course of plasmoquine treatment, following medication for curing an attack, should be advocated as tending to reduces the chance of infection being conveyed to mosquitoes.

ANTI-MALARIA ORGANISATIONS AT THE CENTRE AND IN THE PROVINCES

In an article entitled "The public health aspect of malaria control" in the *Indian Medical Gazette* of December 1942, Major-General G. Covell, I.M.S., Director, Malaria Institute of India, made the following observations :—

"An essential preliminary to the successful control of malaria in India is the formation of an adequately staffed permanent malaria organisation in each province, the activities of which should be linked up with those of the central organisation of the Government of India".

We fully endorse this view. One of the great defects of the anti-malaria campaign in India during the past 50 years was that it consisted of a series of spasmodic attempts to control the disease. This lack of continuity of effort, accompanied as it often was, by the employment of an organisation was insufficient staff and equipment, has been largely responsible for the inadequacy of the results achieved. As we have already said, it has been amply demonstrated, during the present War, that with adequate measures, even the highly malarious regions of the Tropics can be rendered comparatively safe from this disease. Again we have pointed out, in our review of existing conditions, how the malaria organisation, which has been working in the Delhi urban area for the past seven or eight years, has shown that, under civil conditions also a reasonably effective control of the incidence of the disease can be achieved provided adequate funds are expended under the best available technical advice. In these circumstances, we feel that there can be no excuse for Governments in this country not attempting to organise an effective campaign against the disease. Its wide prevalence, the cost involved and the existing inadequacy of trained personnel may result in this campaign being extended over perhaps many years. Even so, it is most important that a beginning should be made and, in the following paragraphs, specific proposals are made towards this end.

Central Malaria Organisation. The Malaria Institute of India is the central organisation for advising the Government of India on all matters relating to this disease as well as for assisting Provincial Governments with such technical advice as they may require. Its functions have been defined by the Director of Malaria Institute in the following terms :—

"1. To be fully informed upon all malaria problems. To advise Government on all issues relative to malaria in India.

2. To initiate enquiries and investigations on malaria. To carry out such enquiries as Government may for any reason require. To assist provincial organisations in the carrying out of such enquiries as may be undertaken by them, providing such assistance as desired and even, in certain cases when thought necessary, to lend officers temporarily from the staff to work under local government.

3. To undertake systematic research in due course into all the basic facts underlying malaria transmission, prevalence and prevention, such as the study of mosquitoes, systematic and bionomical, types of

malaria parasites, transmission power of different species of Anopheles, mechanism of infection including the study of endemic and epidemic phenomena, etc. Gradually to complete and organise knowledge on these subjects and to arrange for the making of such knowledge available for practical application, or such other uses as may be desirable.

4. To carry out epidemiological investigations—mapping of endemicity, study of hyperendemic and healthy areas, study of malaria statistics on modern lines—and generally to elucidate the underlying principles of malaria prevalence in India.

5. To advise upon and assist in the carrying out of anti-malaria measures. To study these scientifically and to judge and elucidate their results.

6. To undertake clinical work on malaria, including treatment. To study serum reactions and allied aids to diagnosis and understanding the disease. To study relapse problems, effects of new drugs, etc.

7. To assist affiliated researches (*e.g.*, kalaazar, filariasis, sandfly fever, dengue, Stegomyia work) by identification of material, provision of trained staff and subordinate personnel.

8. To teach and train officers and others in practical malaria work.

9. To publish scientific results, useful guides, bulletins, etc.

10. To keep alive interest in malaria study and prevention and to see that such interest wherever present is nursed and assisted".

We are in full agreement with the Director that these should be the main function of the Malaria Institute of India.

The permanent establishment of the Institute consists of a Director, an Assistant Director, an Entomologist, an Assistant to the Director, a Malaria Assistant and appropriate subordinate staff. The new posts of a Deputy Director, an Assistant Director and of certain subordinate staff, which were recently created as a temporary measure for the duration of the war, should be made permanent. In view of the large developments that are likely to take place in the activities of this malaria organisation, the Central Health Department should bear in mind the importance of ensuring that it is adequately staffed.

The provincial malaria organisation. The general plan should be the creation of an organisation at the headquarters of each province and, in addition, a number of malaria control units to operate in malarious areas in the districts. The number of these units will obviously depend upon the size of the province and the extent and degree of the prevalence of malaria in it. As an illustration, we may set out a plan for the province of Bengal. We think that about 150 such units will eventually be required for that province, but a beginning may be made with ten. Others can be added as and when additional trained staff and funds become available. But it is essential that, even from the beginning, suitable transport should be provided for these control units in order to increase their mobility, and effectiveness.

In the larger provinces it will be necessary to provide regional organisations also in order to ensure that adequate supervision is exercised over the peripheral malaria control units. In the smaller provinces, however, such regional organisations may not be necessary. Here the Provincial Malaria Officers and their staff should be able to carry out the necessary supervision. This Provincial Officer should have the status of an Assistant Director of Health Services, and the Regional Malaria Officers may be designated Deputy Malaria Officers.

The complete organisation for a large province such as Bengal, may be developed on the following lines :—

1. Provincial Headquarters—

Provincial Malaria Officer	1
Entomologist	1

	Sanitary Engineer	1
	Overseers	4
	Draftsman	1
	Antimalaria Officer	1
	Antimalaria Assistants	2
	Laboratory Assistants	5
	Insect Collectors	8
2.	Deputy Malaria Officers	5
3.	Malaria Control Units—	
	Antimalaria Assistant	1
	Laboratory Assistants	2
	Malaria Supervisors	5
	Fitter Mistri	1
	Field Workers	25

Antimalarial fleld workers are semi-skilled labourers and should not be considered as coolies.

Lists of suitable equipment for the malaria organisation at the provincial headquarters and for the malaria control units are given in Appendix 14 of Volume III* of the report.

These estimates of the malaria organisation desirable for a province such as Bengal, including staff and equipment, were prepared for us by the Director of the Malaria Institute of India. He has suggested the following approximate number of malaria control units for the different provinces.

	No. of control units
Madras	100
Bombay	60
Bengal	150
United Provinces	150
Punjab	60
Bihar	100
Orissa	50

*Appendix A (*a*).

Central Provinces & Berar	100
Assam	80
N. W. F. Province	30
Sind	60
Ajmer-Merwara	5
Baluchistan	30
Delhi Province	2
Coorg	5
	982

He has stated that, in calculating these requirements, he took into account such factors, in respect of each province, as the area, population, number of districts, number of villages and the degree of prevalence of malaria as indicated by (*a*) statistics of malaria mortality, and (*b*) the percentage of fever cases on total cases treated at hospitals and dispensaries.

In our view, the most essential requirements are adequately trained personnel in sufficient numbers and the drugs, appliances and other equipment for carrying on effectively the campaign against the disease. We would, as a general rule, deprecate the spending of large sums on the erection of elaborate buildings in the early stages of our programme for, we believe that such money as is likely to be available can, at the beginning, be much more effectively used on staff and antimalarial measures.

We once again feel it necessary to stress the inestimable value of good rural communications in increasing the effectiveness of all health and other workers employed on nation building tasks in such areas.

For details regarding the staff required for such an organisation reference may be made to Appendix 14. The total expenditure involved in the development of malaria organisations in the Provinces and at the Centre, on the lines suggested by us, during the first five and the second five years of our short-term programme will be as under :—

	Non-recurring expenditure Lakhs	*Recurring expenditure Crores (Rs.)*
First five years	9.17	2.52
Second five years	11.10	3.85

These estimates have been made on the assumption that, during the first five years of the programme, the average number of malaria control units which will be established in individual Governors' Provinces will be 10 and that, during the next five years, fifteen more such units will be added in each province. For each of the Centrally Administered Areas the corresponding number of units proposed is five for each quinquennium.

PROVISION FOR THE HOSPITALISATION OF MALARIA PATIENTS

When our short-term programme for the first ten years has been completed, provision for hospital accommodation for all classes of patients for the country, as a whole, should consist of (1) 30 bed hospitals for every group of two primary units, (2) 216 hospitals with 200 beds each, and (3) 139 hospitals with a bed strength of 500 each in addition to the existing hospitals. While in the small 30 bed hospitals it wil be difficult to allocate special beds for malaria, we have recommended the reservation of 10 and 25 beds respectively for this disease in the 200 and 500 bed hospitals. Thus the number of beds available for the treatment of malaria will be, at the end of the ten year period, a little over 5,600.

By the time our long-term programme is reached such provision for malaria should have increased to the extent shown below :—

Primary unit hospitals	*Secondary unit hospitals*	*District headquarter hospitals*	*Total*
112,500	6,250	2,500	121,250

The number of primary units, by the time this stage is

reached, is likely to be in the neighbourhood of 18,500 to 19,000. Each primary unit hospital will provide six beds for this disease, and in view of the wide distribution of these units, provision for hospitalising such patients will be spread throughout the country. In addition 10 and 20 beds, respectively, have been provided for malaria patients in the hospitals located at the headquarters of secondary units, which will generally correspond to the headquarters of a sub division, and at the district headquarters respectively.

We trust, however, that before this stage is reached, effective and persistent antimalaria measures will have resulted in materially reducing the need for hospital treatment for sufferers from malaria.

THE TRAINING OF MALARIA PERSONNEL

It is anticipated that a certain proportion of the trained personnel of the antimalaria organisation at present employed in the Army will become available for the development of the civil malaria establishments in the provinces after demobilisation. Nevertheless, in the immediate post-war period it will be necessary to train a large number of medical officers in order to fill such posts as those of the Provincial and Deputy Malaria Officers, Officers in charge of control units, Entomologists and Malaria Engineers. We recommend that the training of these types of personnel should, in the immediate post-war period, be carried out in the Malaria Institute of India. It seems to us essential that the development of antimalaria activities in the provinces should be promoted on fairly uniform lines and that the training of these higher types of malaria personnel should, therefore, be carried out at the Malaria Institute of India for some time to come.

On the other hand, the training of overseers, technicians and inspectors or supervisors can be carried out by the Provincial Malaria Organisations in those provinces which have well-developed malaria establishments, namely, Bombay, Madras, the United Provinces, Bengal and Assam. Until the remaining provinces develop similar organisations, the requirements of the Punjab, the N. W. F. Province and Sind can be met by making provision for the training, every year, of a certain number of these types of personnel at the Malaria Institute of India, Delhi. Other provinces can perhaps secure similar facilities by negotiation with the neighbouring provinces where the training of such malaria workers will be developed to meet their own requirements.

It will be seen that the training facilities to be provided at the main Institute at Delhi will thus be considerable. These training functions will necessitate the strengthening of the staff of the Institute beyond the additions suggested by us earlier in this chapter. We recommend that the Central Health Department should take immediate steps to investigate and determine what further strengthening of the establishment will be necessary in order to provide the training facilities the post-war health programmes will require.

We think that the officers of the antimalaria organisations in the provinces should be able to train locally types of workers such as laboratory assistants and attendants, insect collectors, etc.

We wish to make it clear that these recommendations of ours for concentrating the training of the higher types of malaria personnel at Delhi are of a purely temporary nature. When the antimalaria organisations in the provinces become fully developed the provision of training facilities for all types of malaria workers should, in our view, be the responsibility of Provincial Governments. We have suggested, later in this chapter, the creation of Chairs of Malariology in selected medical colleges in order to provide facilities for undergraduate and postgraduate training in the subject as well as for stimulating research. Thus the provinces should, in due course, develop facilities for the highest type of training that may be required in Malariology.

QUININE AND OTHER DRUGS FOR THE TREATMENT OF MALARIA

We have already referred to the use of quinine and

mepacrine for the treatment of malaria. It is possible that other drugs of greater therapeutic value may also be discovered as the result of scientific research. It is, therefore, not easy to estimate accurately what levels of production in India should be recommended for the immediate future in respect of quinine and mepacrine, in order to ensure that proper treatment facilities are made available to a substantial proportion of the sufferers from malaria. All of us are, however, agreed that it should be the responsibility of Governments, Central and Provincial, to take, in mutual consultation, such steps as are necessary to ensure the production in India of antimalaria drugs in sufficient quantities to meet the requirements of the country within the shortest possible period. We are equally agreed that the country should not again be placed at the mercy of a private monopoly which can control, to its own advantage, the price of these drugs which are essential for the maintenance of the health of the people. Whether, in making adequate provision for these drugs, Governments should themselves undertake extensive programmes of production or whether private enterprise can be relied on to supply the needs of the country through any system of guarantees or subsidies from the State, are matters on which we are unable to express an opinion with the information at our disposal. We can only lay down three general propositions :

(1) the prices at which antimalaria drugs are made available to the people should be sufficiently low to enable the poorest classes to obtain them in adequate amounts for the effective treatment of the disease ;

(2) these drugs, in whatever provinces they may be produced, should be made available, on an equitable basis and on reasonable terms, for the needs of all parts of the country ; and

(3) no delay should be allowed to occur in developing their production.

We shall first consider the production of quinine.

(*a*) *Quinine.* If Colonel Sinton's estimate that at least

one hundred million individuals suffer from the disease every year be taken as the basis of calculation, it does not seem unreasonable to assume that there will be at least 120 to 150 million cases to be treated annually in view of the fact that more than one attack is not an uncommon feature of the disease. The Malaria Commission has recommended 75 grains of quinine as the minimum quantity necessary for the treatment of a case On this basis the amount of quinine required will be in the neighbourhood of 1.3 to 1.6 million pounds per year. If quinine is to be relied upon as the sole durg for the treatment of malaria our objective should be an annual production of it to the extent of about 1.5 million pounds from cinchona bark produced in the country. Some of us hold the view that this should be the definite objective which Governments should place before themselves and that every endeavour should be made to attain it within the shortest period that may be practicable. Others feel that the experience gained during the War with the large scale use of mepacrine in the treatment and prevention of malaria in highly endemic areas, makes it necessary to take into account the possibility of this drug replacing quinine to a greater or less extent in the treatment of the disease and that it would, in the circumstances, be safer to start with a more limited objective in regard to the production of quinine. The average annual consumption of quinine in India in the pre-war period was 210,000 lbs. and, of this amount, about a third was produced in India, a part of such production being, we believe, from bark imported from Java. As a practical objective for realisation as early as possible those of us who hold this view recommend the raising of quinine production to the pre-war level of consumption in India, namely, about 210,000 lbs. from indigenous bark alone. A cinchona plant begins to yield bark generally from the fifth year of its life, the period of high productivity being from the fifth to the ninth year. After the twelfth year its yield gradually decreases. In these circumstances the raising of the annual production of quinine even to 210,000 lbs. mark from bark produced in the country will take some years. In the meantime the possibility of synthetic drugs displacing quinine, wholly or in part, in the treatment of malaria may well be settled. This is a question of considerable importance which should be decided before embarking on too ambitious a programme of quinine production. Such a programme is certain to involve heavy financial commitments which would not be justified if it became possible to produce cheaper and equally effective synthetic substitutes.

We, as a committee, would prefer to leave to the Governments in the country the responsibility for deciding whether private enterprise should or should not be associated with the production of quinine and of other antimalaria drugs. If it is decided that such association is desirable it would be for Governments to determine the conditions under which private agencies should participate in production. One of us (Sir Frederick James), however, desires to see that private agencies are given the fullest opportunity to take part in quinine production with technical advice and a price guarantee provided by the State. We attach our colleague's note on the subject. We fully support his suggestion that research into the agricultural and manufacturing aspects of the quinine industry should be a governmental resposibility and that two experimental stations should be established to serve North and South India respectively.

(*b*) *Mepacrine.* The pre-war annual consumption figure of 210,000 lbs. of quinine will provide treatment, at the rate of 75 grains per patient, for about 19.6 or nearly 20 million cases of malaria. If, as an immediate objective, we accept the provision of adequate antimalaria drugs for the treatment of 50 million cases annually, then sufficient mepacrine will have to be produced to meet the requirements of 30 million patients. The minimum quantity of this drugs for a complete course for a patient is 1.5 grammes or 15 tablets of 0.1 gramme each. The manufacture of 450 million tablets of mepacrine a year in India should, therefore, be the immediate objective.

Pyrethrum and D.D.T. The main sources of pyrethrum, before the War, were Kenya and Japan but the cultivation of the plant has been successfully undertaken in various parts of India, including Kashmir, the Punjab Hills, the U.P., Central Provinces, Madras and Orissa. It has been shown that the yield of the active principle from the plants, grown in many parts of India, compares favourably with the flowers obtained from Kenya. In these circumstances, it may be reasonably expected that, in the course of some years, there will be an ample supply of pyrethrum grown in this country, to meet all local demands. The Director, Malaria Institute of India, has estimated that, in order to make the country self-sufficient, pyrethrum cultivation will have to be extended to about 120,000 acres so as to produce annually about 15,000 short tons (2,000 lbs. a ton) of pyrethrum flowers. This estimate makes allowance for a sixth of the total area under cultivation lying fallow each year.

As an insecticide the relationship of D.D.T. to pyrethrum is somewhat similar to that of mepacrine to quinine in the treatment of malaria. There is the possibility, in both cases, of the synthetic substance replacing, to a greater or less extent, the use of the other. It may, however, be pointed out that the indiscriminate use of D.D.T. has been shown to result in the destruction of cerain types of beneficial insects. It is quite likely that, in due course, adequate safeguards will be discovered and introduced in order to prevent these detrimental effects. There is also the possibility that insecticides more potent than D.D.T. may be produced and brought into use. While recognising that these possibilities should be given due weight, we think that, the cultivation of pyrethrum in India should be developed until the use of D.D.T. has become established. Even when this stage is reached, the production of a certain amount of pyrethrum will still be necessary, if as has been suggested a combination of D.D.T. and pyrethrum is more effective than either of them alone. Another reason which has prompted us to advocate the continuance of its cultivation is that at short notice, it can, if necessary, be given up and replaced by other crops. Here again the steps required to foster the increased growth of pyrethrum must be decided by Governments after a full examination of the relevant factors.

We can only stress the necessity for a largely increased

supply of pyrethrum flowers at a reasonable price and the duty of Governments in India to take immediate steps to ensure production on a scale sufficient for the needs of the country.

Clinical Research in Malaria. While one line of attack in the malaria problem is through the control of the carrier types of mosquitoes, another should be directed towards the elimination of the reservoirs of infection. As relapses are quite common in malaria, a person who suffers from an attack of the disease continues, in an appreciable percentage of cases, to harbour the parasite for a varying length of time. The complete destruction of all the parasites in such persons should form an important part of an antimalarial campaign. One of the limitations of all antimalarial drugs so far available (including quinine, mepacrine and plasmoquine) is that they help to kill only such of the parasites as are present in the circulating blood of the patient while those which are harboured in the spleen and other internal organs escape. The achievements of chemotherapy have, during recent years, been so brilliant that it is quite conceivable that a drug may be discovered with power to kill the parasite not only in the circulating blood but also in those internal organs in which it finds refuge. Any such drug when discovered and tested in the laboratory can be considered to be effective only by a reasonably large field trial on human beings. We feel that there is need for the active promotion of combined biochemical and clinical research aiming at the evolution of a suitable drug which will help not only to cure patient for the time being, but also to destroy the parasites in him completely.

We consider the promotion of active research in malaria to be of fundamental importance in this country. The creation of Chairs of Malariology in selected medical colleges is a highly desirable step in this connection. These professorships would serve a double purpose, namely, the fostering of research in malaria and the provision of adequate facilities for undergraduate and postgraduate training in the subject.

Legislation. The effective enforcement of antimosquito

measures requires suitable legislation and we have given, as appendices 15, 16 and 17 respectively, the Model Mosquito Ordinance of the United States Public Health Service, the Straits Settlements Destruction of Mosquitoes Ordinance No. 174 and those sections of the Bombay City Municipal Act which deal with antimosquito measures, in order that they may be examined by the different health authorities in the country with a view to seeing how far they may be followed as models.

CERTAIN SUGGESTIONS BY SIR FREDERICK JAMES, O.B.E., M.L.A., FOR INCREASING QUININE PRODUCTION

(1) Before deciding on the method of increasing the production of cinchona bark in India it would be well to study the production methods in the Netherlands East Indies which, before the War, supplied over 90 per cent of the world's quinine. Their dominating position has been achieved through a combination of Government and private efforts and the systematic way in which the industry has been organised.

(2) Nine-tenths of the cinchona produced in the N.E. Indies comes from private plantations, but the improved types of cinchona and the improved methods of cultivation and propagation are derived from the work carried out at the Government cinchona plantations. Judged by ordinary standards of commercial accountancy the production of cinchona on private estates will always be cheaper than on Government estates. If, therefore, the aim is to produce quinine at as reasonable a cost as possible, every attempt should be made to persuade planters to take up its cultivation.

(3) A Central Cinchona Bureau for India similar to the Kina Bureau of the Netherlands East Indies should be established. Such a Bureau might well have two experimental stations, one situated in the North and the other situated in the South with plantations attached. If such a Bureau were placed under the Imperial Council of Agricultural Research, and private planters were associated with it, India would have taken the first step towards raising cheap cinchona, for the only

bark which is really cheap is the bark of the high yielding types.

(4) The main work on both these experimental stations would be the study of plant breeding, vegetative propagation, cultivation, manuring and the regeneration of plantations, which had already finished one cycle of cinchona growing.

(5) One of the reasons why cinchona production has been so backward in India is its provincialization in Madras and Bengal, the lack of an all-India policy, and the failure of the Governments concerned either to associate experienced planters with the development of their stations or to encourage private enterprise.

(6) On page 153 there are two general propositions :—

(*a*) 'That the prices at which antimalaria drugs, including quinine, are made available to the people should be sufficiently low to enable the poorest classes to obtain them in adequate amounts for the effective treatment of the disease'. This will involve a certain amount of price control and, in the event of private plantations being encouraged, profit control also. But the planting of cinchona is a risky enterprise and if profits are to be controlled in order to ensure that the price of quinine is kept at a reasonably low level, then a guaranteed offtake at a fixed price is the only inducement which will encourage private enterprise. The world price of cinchona has fluctuated around Rs. 20 per lb. and the experience of the Netherlands East Indies has shown that a reasonably profitable industry can be a sound basis for a normal and constant production. This should be recognised by those who wish to see quinine provided at a cheap price, for it can only be achieved if economy is effected in the costs of production and distribution by efficient management, or funds are provided from public revenues to meet the loss incurred by inefficient production. Costs of production can be reduced by scientific research and efficient organisation, and of this, industry is well aware.

(*b*) That no delay should be allowed to occur in starting new plantations on an adequate scale. If a Central Cinchona Bureau is established, it should be fairly simple to plan production with a view both to ensuring supplies of bark to existing factories and where new areas are being opened up for the maintenance of other factories in full production.

Government stations should also assist by raising plants of good quality for sale to private growers. Sales would be partly adjusted to the cinchona which they desired to establish in any areas.

The cinchona industry should be essentially an all-India concern, but at present it is provincial and dealt with by two provincial Governments. If the price guarantee is agreed to by the Central Government, then it could be made conditional on a certain amount of control over policy, both of extensions and scientific research. If the Madras and the Bengal Governments are not prepared to associate the Imperial Council of Agricultural Research with the planning of the work at their stations, then the Central Government should establish its own research station in Coorg which is a centrally administered area and is suitable for plantation of cinchona.

APPENDIX A (*a*)

PROVINCIAL MALARIA ORGANISATION

(*a*) Provincial Headquarters staff :

	First Five years	Second five years
Assistant Director of Health Services (Malariology)	1	
Entomologist	1	
Sanitary Engineer	1	
Overseers	4	
Draftsman	1	
Antimalaria Officer	1	The same staff
Laboratory Assistants	5	
Antimalaria Assistants... ...	2	
Clerks	3	
Insect collectors	8	
Inferior servants	2	
Sweepers	2	

(*b*) Regional Organisations—While five Deputy Assistant Directors are eventually to be provided in all the major provinces none will be appointed during the first five years and only two such posts will be created during the second five years.

First Five years	Second five years
Nil	Deputy Assistant Directors of Health ... 2
	Clerks ... 2

(*c*) Malaria Con trol Units :

Staff on one units :—		First five years	Second five years
		Number of malaria control units to be established during the	
Antimalaria assistant	1		
Laboratory assistants	2		
Malaria Supervisors	5	10	15
Mistry	1		
Field worker ...	25		

List of equipment required for the Provincial Headquarters Unit

1. Microscopes, high power ... ... Ten
2. Microscopes, dissecting, small ... Ten
3. Microscopes, dissecting, binocular ... Two
4. Other laboratory equipment of the type of hand lenses, breeding cages, glassware balance, primus stoves, etc., including chemicals ... — ... As required (A yearly allotment of Rs. 800)
5. Surveyor's equipment for the Sanitary Engineer and his staff
6. Bicycles ... — ... Ten
7. Typewriters, standard ... ... Two
8. Typewriters, portable ... ... One
9. Epidiascope for instructional purposes One
10. Cinema Projector instructional purposes One

List of equipment required for the Provincial Control Unit

(*a*) Transport—

(1) Trucks, 3/4 ton 4×4, weapons carrier Two
(2) Trucks, 3/4 ton, 4×4 (Jeep) ... One

(*b*) Tentage—

Tents, 160 pound ... ... Three

(*c*) Sprayers, spraying equipment, etc.—

(1) Petrol driven sprayers, 1 to 2 H.P.... Four

(2) MISH type hand sprayers ... One hundred

(3) Knapsack sprayers, oil ... ... Twelve

(4) Stirrup pumps, double barrel, complete with special nozzles, lenses, etc. Twenty

(5) Empty drums, 40 gallons Five

(6) Empty drums, 5 gallons... ... Twenty

(7) Empty drums, 1 gallon ... ... Twenty

(8) Buckets 3—4 gallons ... ... Forty

(*d*) Field Worker's Implements—

(1) Hoes ... ... Two dozen

(2) Pick axes ... ... One dozen

(3) Matchets ... ... Two dozen

(4) Axes, wood cutting ... ... Six

(*e*) Laboratory equipment such as hand lenses, breeding cages, catching apparatus, glassware, balance, primus stoves, etc.... As required (A yearly allotment of Rs. 3,000)

(*f*) Portable typewriter ... ... One

APPENDIX B

A NOTE ON MALARIA IN ANCIENT INDIA*

The texts of verses on fever and malaria in *the Athurva Veda* (1500 B.C.) the *Caraka Samhita* (c300 B.C.) and *the Susruta Samhita* (c100 B.C.) with their translation in English and extracts from accounts of travels of Marco Polo, the Italian traveller (born in Venice) are given in this note.

Although Marco Polo visited India (Kayal in Tamraparni) in 1288 and 1293 A.D., the use of mosquito-nets described by him may be an ancient practice.

FEVER IN ATHARVA-VEDA

The word *takman* (तक्मन्) was used for fever in *Atharva-veda.* During the *Ayurvedic* period the word *jwara* (ज्वर) was introduced.

The *takman* or *jwara* is used for all kinds of fever. It was a group name and not meant for malarial fever exclusively. It included typhoid group, puerperal group, pneumonia group, tuberculosis group, and all other groups of fever. Malaria being the commonest type of fever, a large number of references are found relating to malaria. The malarial type was—common in a country where there was abundance of rain (महावृषः) or where there was too much of grass (मूजः).

It was classified in *Atharvavedic* period as quotidian (सदन्दि) tertian (तृतीयकम्) and quartan (वितृतीयम्). It was also classified according to the season in which the fever made its appearance,

*The valuable advice of Dr. Pranjivan Manekchand Mehta is gratefully acknowledged.

namely, (शीतम्) (winter), (ग्रैष्मम्) (summer), वार्षिकम् (rainy season).

ये शालाः परि नृत्यन्ति सायं गर्दभनादिनः ।
कुसूला ये च कुक्षिलाः ककुभाः करुभाः स्रिमाः ।
तानोषधे त्वं गन्धेन विषूचीनान् विनाशय ॥ १० ॥

अथर्ववेद का ८, सू. ६

They who dance round the dwellings in the evening, making loud braying—like noises—they that are provided with needle like—probscis, large bellies, and humped backs and which are grotesque and make evil noises—these, 0 herb, with thy smell do thou make to—disappear scattered.

ये कुकुन्धाः कुकूरभाः कृत्तीर्दूर्शानि बिभ्रति ।
क्लीवा इव प्रनृत्यन्तो वने ये कुर्वते घोषं तानितो नाशयामसि ॥ ११ ॥

The Kukundhas, the Kukurabhas, that bear skins, pelts, dancing on like impotent men, that make a noise in the forest—them we make disappear from here.

ये सूर्यं न तितिक्षन्त आतपन्तममुं दिवः ।
अरायान् बस्ति वासिनो दुर्गन्धी क्लोहितास्यान् मक्कान् नाशयामसि ॥ १२ ॥

They who do not endure yonder sun, burning down from the sky, the niggard bleaters, ill-smelling, bloody mouthed, the mosquitoes, we make to disapear.

ये सूर्यात् परिसर्पन्ति स्नुषेव श्वसुरादधि ।
बजस्र्वव तेषां पिङ्गश्व हृदयेऽधि नि विध्यतान् ॥२४ ॥

They that creep away from the sun, as a daughter-in-law away from the father-in-law—let the drugs *Baja* and *Pinga* pierce into their heart.

तक्मन् भ्रात्रा बालासेन रचस्रा कासिकया सह ।
पाप्मा भ्रातृव्येण सह गच्छामुमरणं जनम् ॥ १२ ॥
तृतीयकं वितृतीयं सदन्दिमुत शारदम् ।
तक्मानं शीतं रूरं ग्रैष्मं नाशय वार्षिकम् ॥ १३ ॥

गन्धारिभ्यो मूजवदभ्योऽङ्गेभ्यो मगधेभ्यः ।
प्रैष्यन् जनमिव शेवधिं तक्मानं परिदद्मसि।। १४ ।।
अथर्ववेद का, ५ सू० २२

O fever, together with thy brother the *Balasa* (and) thy sister the cough, together with thy cousin the scab (*Papman*) go to yon foreign people.

The fever of the third day, of two days out of three, the constant and the autumnal, the cold, the hot, that of the hot season, that of the reainy season, do thou cause to disappear.

To the *Gandharis**, the *Majavants, the Angas**, *the Magadhas**, like one sending a person a treasure, do we commit the fever.

ओको अस्य मूजवन्त ओको अस्य महावृषाः ।
यावज्जातस्तकमं स्तावानसि बह्लिकेषु न्योचरः ।। ५ ।।

Its home (*Okas*) is the (*Mujavants*), its home is the *Mahavrsa*, as long as born, O fever, so long art thou at home among the *Bahlikas.**

**Gandhara*—The country of Gandhara lies along the Kabul river between the Khoaspes (Kunar) and the Indus. Its capital was Purusapura, now called Peshawar......

Gandhara comprised the districts of Peshawar and Hotimurdan or what is called the Eusofzai country. *Anga*—The country about Bhagalpur in Bengal. Its capital was Champapuri. Its western boundary was the junction of the Ganges and the Taraju. It was the kingdom of Karna of the Mahabharata. *Balkh* (Vahlika : Bactriana of the Greeks). *Bahlikas*—Always associated with the people of the north, west and ultra-Indian provinces, and usually considered to represent the Bactrians or people of Balkh. *Magadha*—The province of Bihar. Its western boundary was the river Sona. The ancient capital of Magadha was Girivrajapura (modern Rajgir) at the time of Jarasandha who was killed by Bhima, one of the 5 Pandavas. The capital was subsequently removed to Pataliputra, which was formerly an insignificant village called by the name of Patligrama, enlarged and strengthend by Ajatasatru, king of Magadha and contemporary of Buddha.........At one period, the country of Magadha extended south of the Ganges from Benares to Monghir and southwards as far as Singhbum.

The description of the flying insect gives nearly all the characteristics of the form and life of the mosquito and also of fragrant or fumigating medications used to destroy the mosquitoes. The word used is मक्क which is equal to मशक: in classical Sanskrit. The derivatives of the word mosquito in different languages are as under :—

Greek : μvia=fly. Latin : Musca, a fly. Sanskrit : मशक: a mosquito मश् : to hum buzz to make a noise.

All derivatives suggest the common origin ; hence the word must have originated before the two Aryan groups migrated to other lands, one to Greece and the other to India, *i.e.*, before the formation of Sanskrit or Greek language ; hence both the languages have common term as the source of the word.

FEVER IN CARAKA AND SUSRUTA, SAMHITAS

The word *takman* replaced by the word *jwara* (ज्वर :) continues to be the group-name of all diseases with fever as the main and dominating sign, Caraka and Susruta classify fever in five types instead of four of the *Atharva-Veda*.

They are : संतत: = Continuous. सतत: = Remittent. अन्येद्युष्क: = Quotidian. तृतीयक: = Tertian and चतुर्थक: = Quartan.

Fever was considered the most dreadful of diseases. The simili given in *Caraka Samhita* to explain the advent and periodicity of this kind of fever is interesting. Caraka compares the phenomena to the seed sown in the ground which grows up at a particular time ; Malaria causative factor is like a seed which takes one day to grow in case of quotidian, two days in case of tertian and three days in case of quartan. When "the seed" grow up, they invade the whole body and not being counteracted by anti-bodies, (प्रत्यनीक), they cause the fever. When the force of these invading elements is exhausted, they return to their original habitat and again begin to grow up. The simili given by Caraka closely reflects our present knowledge of the life history of malaria parasite.

Sushruta compares the advent of fever to the tide and ebb of the ocean.

Both the authors state that this kind of fever is common in low land or land at the foot of the mountain.

Caraka

पुनः पञ्चविधो दृष्टो दोषकाल बलाबलात् ।
संततः सततोऽन्येद्युस्तृतीयक चतुर्थकौ ॥

च. चि. ३, ३४

Again, fever is seem to be of five kinds viewed in the light of the strength or weakness of the morbific factor and the season ; thus it is continuous, intermittent, quotidian, tertian and quartan.

अहोरात्रे सततको द्वौ कालावनुवर्तते ।

Remittent fever which periodically rising and remitting has two phases of rise of fever in one day.

अन्येद्युष्कः प्रतिदिनं दिनं हित्वा तृतीयकः ।
दिनद्वयं यो विश्रम्य प्रत्येति स चतुर्थकः ॥

च. चि. ३, ६७

The quotidian fever recurs everyday, the tertian fever with an interval of a day and that is quartan fever which recurs with an interval of two days.

अधिशेते यथा भूमिं बीजं काले च रोहति ।
अधिशेते तथा धातु दोषः काले च कुप्यति ॥
स वृद्धि बलकालं च प्राप्य दोषस्तृतीयकम् ।
चतुर्थकं च कुरुते प्रत्यनीक बलक्षयात् ॥
कृत्वा वेगं गतबलाः स्वे स्वे स्थाने व्यवस्थिताः ।
पुनर्विवृद्धाः स्वे काले ज्वरयन्ति नरं मलाः ॥

च. चि. ३, ६८-६९-७०

Just as the seed lies dormant in the soil and germinates in season, in the same manner the toxic matter lies into quiescence in the body-element and flares up when the time is ripe.

Thus the morbific factor gathering strength and biding the propitious time, manifests itself as the tertian or the quartan fever as soon as the disease-resisting power in the body is lowered.

In this manner, the disease-generating factors, having worked themselves out, lapse into quiescence and retire to their respective stations in the body ; then mustering up their strength, once again, these toxic elements afflict the patient with fever at their own ripe times.

Susruta

सप्ताहं वा दशाह वा द्वादशाहमथापि वा।
सन्तत्या योऽविसर्गी स्यात्सन्ततः स निगद्यते ॥
अहोरात्रे सततको द्वौ कालावनुवर्तते।
अन्येद्युष्क स्त्वहोरात्रादेककालं प्रवर्तते ॥
तृतीयक स्तृतीयेऽह्नि चतुर्थेऽह्नि चतुर्थकः।

सु. उ. ३९, ६९-७०-७१

That is called *Santata* fever which persists continually for 7 days, 10 days or even 12 days. The *Santataka* fever repeats twice—during the day and night, while the *Anyedyuska* type arises only once during the day and night. The tertian fever arises on the third day and the quartan on every fourth day.

यथा वेगागमे वेलां छादयित्वा महोदधेः।
वेगहानौ तदेवाम्भस्त त्रैवान्तर्निलीयते ॥
दोषवेगोदये तद्वदुदीर्येत ज्वरोऽस्य वै।
वेगहानौ प्रशाम्येत यथाऽम्भः सागरे तथा ॥

सु. उ. ३९, ७३-७४

As the same waters of the ocean having covered the sea-coast at the time of high tide again hide themselves inside at the very place at the ebbing time, in the same way fever springs up at the time of the rise of the strength of the provoked humors and again subsides with the subsidence of the provocation just as the waters do in the ocean.

औपत्यके मद्यसमुभ्दवे च
हेतुं ज्वरे पित्त्कृतं वदन्ति ।। सु. उ. ३९

Pitta is said to be the etiological factor in the fever of low lands and in that caused by wines.

औपत्यके—पर्वतासन्नभूमिसमुभ्दवे ज्वरे ।
(टीका—उत्त्कृण)

Aupatyaka means—in the fever taking rise in the land just—adjoining the mountains.

उपत्यका—Land at the foot of a hill or mountain; low land.

The mosquitoes (मशक): are classified in five groups by—Sushruta.

मशका: सामुद्रः, परिमण्डलो, हस्तिमशकः, कृष्णः, पार्वतीय इति पञ्च; तैर्दष्टस्य तीव्रा कण्डूर्दंशशोफश्च, पार्वतीयस्तु कीटैः प्राणहरैस्तुल्यलक्षणः ।
सु. क. ८, ३६

The varieties of mosquitoes are five *Samudra* (Sea Born), *Parimandala* (globular in shape), *Hasti-Masaka* (Elephantine type, huge), *Krsna* (Black in colour) and the *Parvaitya* (mountainous species). By their sting there result acute itching and swelling round the sting ; while the bite of the mountainous species bears the characteristics of deadly insects.

VAGBHATA, MADHAVA, BHAVMISRA

Later references by Vagbhata, Madhava and Bhavamishra are simply copied or quoted materials from these two authors. No new references are found. विषम is the irregular type of fever. सम means regular and विषम is irregular.

MARCOPOLO* ON MOSQUITO NETS

The quotation of Yule and also his remark on doubting the correctness of the translation by Marsden (who mixes up mosquito-curtain with a swinging bed) are given here.

"The men of this country have their beds made of very light canework, so arranged that, when they have got in and are going to sleep, they are drawn up by cords nearly to the ceiling and fixed there for the night. This is done to get out of the way of tarantulas which give terrible bites, as well as of fleas and such vermin, and at the same time to get as much air as possible in the great heat which prevails in that region. Not that everybody does this, but only the nobles and great folks, for the others sleep on the streets". (*Travels of Marco Polo*... Vol. II By. Yule. 346).

*Marco Polo (1254 ?-1334 ?) the Venetian, travelled widely to Sivas, Mosul. Baghdad, Hormuz, Khursan to Amu Darya, to the Pamirs, by way of Kashgar, Yarkand and Khotan to Lop Nor, then by way of the Gobi desert to Tangut and Shangu. In 1295, he met Kublai Khan in Shangtu. So far he was accompanying his father and uncle. He then joined diplomatic service of Kublai Khan and visited various parts of the Mongol Empire as Kublai Khan's emissary. He visited India (Kayal on the Tamrapani) in 1288 and also in 1293 on his way back to Venice. On his journey back to Venice from China 1292 besides India he passed through Indonesia, and Persia. At Gena he was imprisoned for one year In 1298. During his imprisonment he dictated the account of his travels, which have been published as the Book of *Marco Polo*. Marco Polo described Kayal in Pandya kingdom as a prosperous city with merchants and foreign traders. He also noticed the use of mosquito-nets by the effluent section of the population. His description of the mosquito-nets, gives the impression that use of such nets was unique to India, not found in other countries visited by him. It may also be conjectured that the mosquito-nets as described by him were in use for considerably long time.

A view was expressed that these were not mosquito-nets but "bed-swings". Such a view has been contradicted by Yule in the above extract.

Note : 19. The first part of this paragraph as rendered by Marsden : "The natives make use of a kind of bedstead or cot of very light canework, so ingenously contrived that when they repose on them, and are inclined to sleep, they can draw close the curtains about them by pulling a string." This is not translation. An approximate illustration of the real statement is found in Pyrard deLaval, who says (of the Maldive Islanders): "Their beds are hung up by four cords to a bar supported by two pillars...The beds of the king, the grandees, and rich folk are made thus that they may be swung and rocked with facility". (Charton, IV. 277). In the Ras Mala swinging cots are several times alluded to. (1.173, 247, 423). In one case the bed is mentioned as suspended to the ceiling by chains. (*Travels of Marco Polo*...Vol II. by Yule, 352.

APPENDIX C

SOME REMINISCENCES OF BIO-ENVIRONMENTAL MEASURES FOR MALARIA CONTROL IN YOL*

Yol Camp, near Dharamsala in Kangra Valley, was built to house the Italian prisoners of war. At the time the camp was built there was an influx of a large labour population. A small part of it continued to live in the outskirts of the camp even after the completion of the camp. The number of civilian population gradually increased to provide varied services to the main population of the camp.

The main population of the camp during 1942-45 varied from about 19000 to about 12000. In early years there were 16,000 Italian prisoners of war (12,000 officers and 4000 other ranks), over 80 British and Indian officers, about 17,00 Indian other ranks and about 250 British other ranks. A Prisoners of War Camp Hospital was built. It had three wings, Italian, Indian and British, virtually a cluster of three hospitals *viz.*, a hospital for prisoners of war with 600 beds ; an Indian Military Hospital with 90 beds ; and a British Military Hospital with a Family Hospital Wing and Camp hygiene and

*The author was posted in Yol Camp from 23.6.41-5.9 1945. Before the camp was built served as medical officer-in-charge mainly to survey the area and advise on measures related to health (water supply, sewrage, plans for disinfestation centre, Prisoner of War Camp Hospital etc.). After establishment of the Prisoner of War Camp Hospital he served for about three years as Second-in Cammand and for a short period as Officer commanding ; through-out this period one of his responsibilities was hygiene and malaria control organisation.

malaria control organisation. The Commanding Officer of the Prisoners of War Camp Hospital was the Senior Executive Medical Officer of the Camp. The direct responsibility of hygiene and malaria control was delegated by him to an officer who was ex-officio Hygiene and Malaria Officer of the Camp.

The Yol Camp was practically surrounded on all sides with rice fields, seepages, and streams. At some distance were houses of handsome, friendly, cheerful and hardworking villagers. Mosquitoes *A. culicifacies*, *A. fluviatilis*, *A. subpictus*, *A. splendidis*, *A. stephensi*, *A. lindsiyi*, *A. gigus* and *A. maculatus* were breeding in abundance in immediate vicinity of the camp and also a little further away from the camp. Dissection of mosquitoes showed *A. fluviatilis* and *A. stephensi* infection rate of 0.9 per cent and 4.5 per cent respectively. *A. culicifacies* was seriously suspected. The mosquito breeding places were posing a serious problem, especially in irrigation channels, ponds, pools, seepages and in a wide expanse of water-logged area. The farmers readily understood the problem, when it was explained to them during discussion, and offered full cooperation and participation in eliminating the breeding places. They wanted an assurance that any measure adopted by them to eliminate mosquito breeding places would not harm their crops and if there was no alternative other than toe use of anti-larval methods harmful to their crops they should recieve written gaurantee as compensation. Such an attitude of the farmers, with very modest income, was understandable. Oiling or any chemical larvicides, therefore, were put aside, except in a very limited area. There were a number of encouraging reports on bio-environmental control of malaria (called naturalistic methods at that time). Their feasibility in Yol was examined. Generally the antilarval measures considered were : clean weeding ; canalising ; flooding, sluicing (hand operated, pipe or pipeless siphons) ; silting ; agitating the surface of water ; alteration of food supply (in Java green algae was replaced by blue-green algae) ; increasing or decreasing the salt content of water ; destroying food supply of the larvae such as by ferrugenous water; deep shading (with hibiscus, melastoma, or lantana) ; and larvivorous fish. Among the naturalistic methods reported for control of malaria there was one which changed the mosquito feeding habit from blood of human beings to that of animals, by placing cowsheds or other animal sheds between mosquito breeding places and human habitation. Mainly three methods were considered feasible for Yol.

SUB-DRAINAGE

For the large water-logged area, it was decided to try "sub-drainge". Broadly it implied digging of open drains and covering them with stones and finally dressing them with earth and grass. All such drains were led to contour drains, which were already in existence and were being used as irrigation channels. Clean weeding was done in these irrigation channels. The water logged area, where there was mosquito breeding on a large scale and walking was practically impossible, was thus converted into lush green grazing ground, free of mosquito breeding places. The report of Mr. V.N. Rao, the Anti-Malaria Assistant, sent by Lt. Colonel K.S. Pillai, I.A.M.C. in October 1949, shows that the sub-drainage required maintenance in that year, *i.e.* for over five years this part of Yol has continued to be free from large scale water collections and free from mosquito breeding ; and with some maintenance the present position is likely to continue.

FLUSHING

In a selected stream, attempts were made to imitate Nature's method of flushing down the larvae. Modified "De Villers siphon" was tried, with the help of Engineering services. This was found to be a simple construction. It required building a wall in the selected site in the stream to get a head of water ; empty drums 22″ diameter, 2′ 11″ high ; concrete pipes 12″ in diameter and galvanised iron pipe 3/4″ diameter.

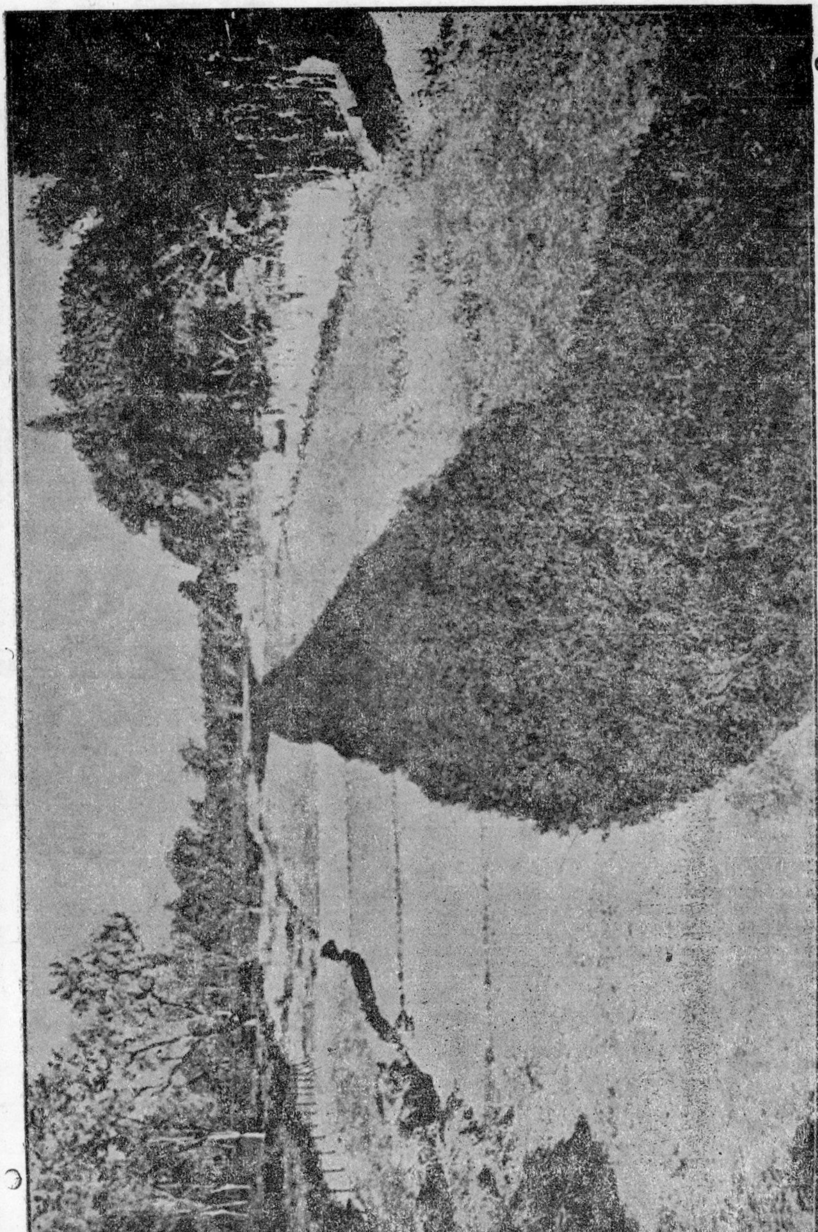

Deep Shading : Anti-Malaria Hedge Lantana considered but found not Feasible for use in Yol

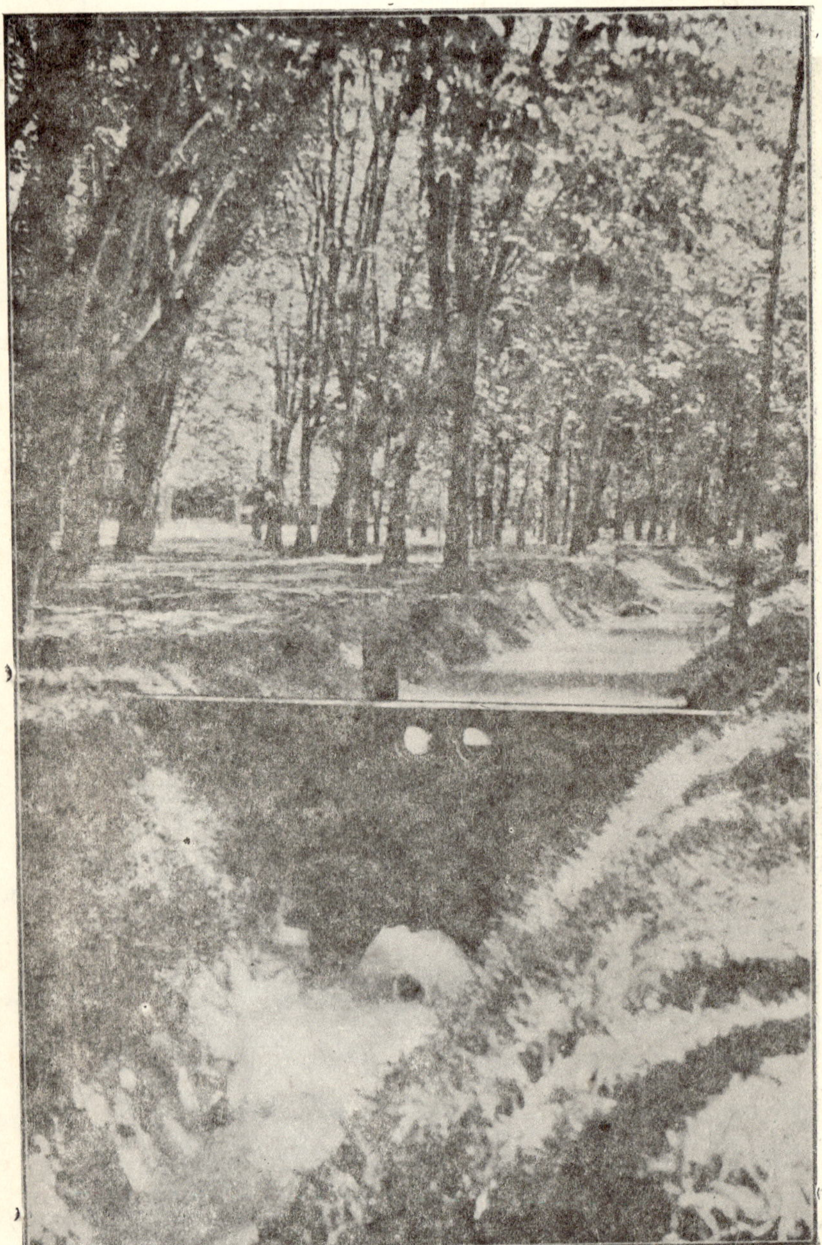

De Viller's Siphon in action successfully nsed in Yol after some modifications

The siphon operate on a simple principle : when the water rises in the catchment area it first flows through 3/4" galvanised iron pipe, sucking air from the drum causing unequal pressure inside and outside the drum, the inequality of pressure starts the flow of water, and when the water level falls and air is able to enter in the inlet the vaccum is destroyed and siphon stops and the cycle re-starts with the rise of water in the catchment area.

Despite the principle of its operation and building of the siphon being simple, several problems were faced. It was found that one siphon didnot effectively flush out the slow running stream and pockets in which mosquitoes were breeding. When two siphons were installed, they didnot operate simultaneously, and also tended to erode the stream bed on the flushing sides of the siphons. The most disappointing experience was damage or destruction of the siphon. During "the natural flooding season the boulders and stones were dislodged and damaged the siphon and with heavy floods the wall at the site of the siphon gave way and the siphon was washed away. This was a distressing but valuable experience and helped to build and use siphon successfully, mainly through paying greater attention to three aspects in building the siphon *viz.* : (*i*) a well selected site free from boulders likely to be dislodged in monsoon ; (*ii*) a good cement concrete wall with overflow pipes and cement flooring of the bed of the stream a few feet beyond the limit where main "flush of the water" falls ; and (*iii*) a pipe connecting the drums at the top to synchronise the action of two siphons.

After the above changes were made the siphon functioned satisfactorily and mosquito breeding along this stream was eliminated. According to the report of Mr. V.N. Rao, Anti-malaria Assistant of 1949, referred above, the siphon worked satisfactorily and till 1946 the concrete damn was in fairly good condition. After 1946, it did not work satisfactorily, due to inability to carry out maintenance in the period when the camp remained closed, stream water percolated through stones and

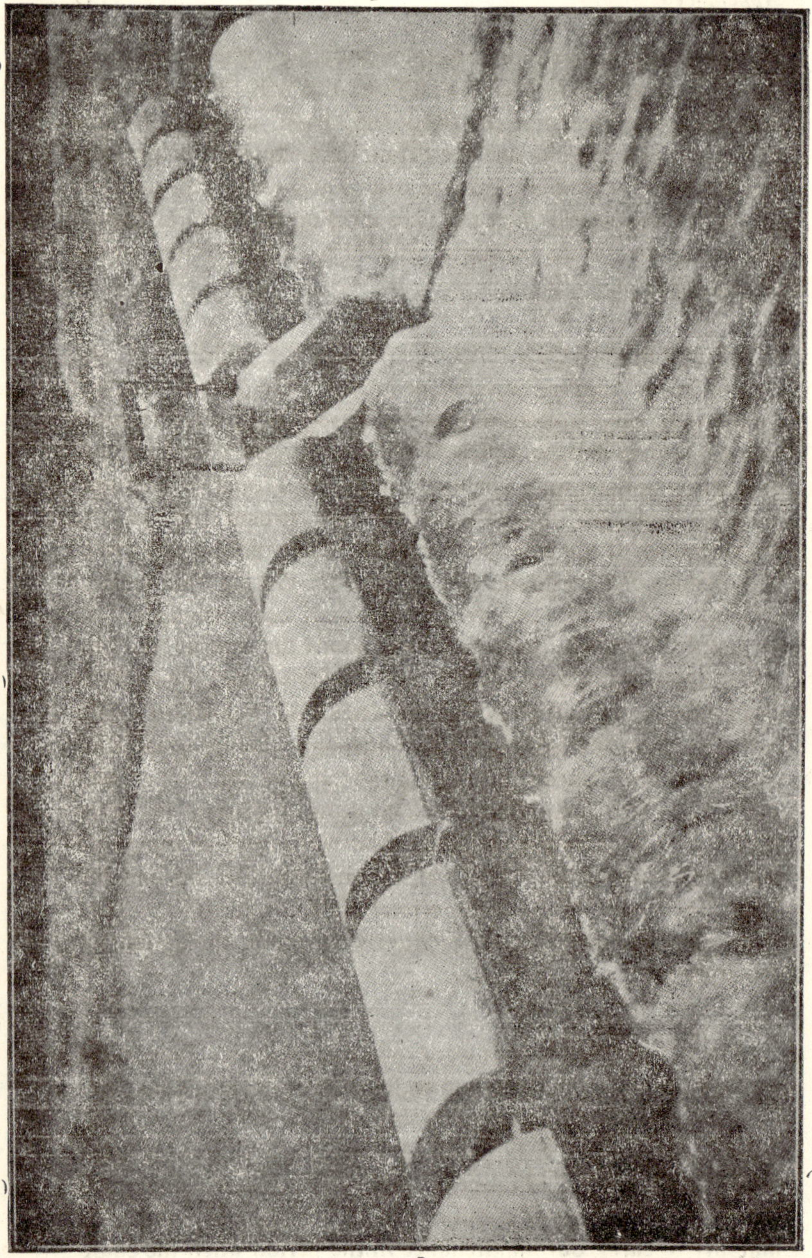

Battery of Automatic Siphons in Action. A Battery of two De Ville's Siphons

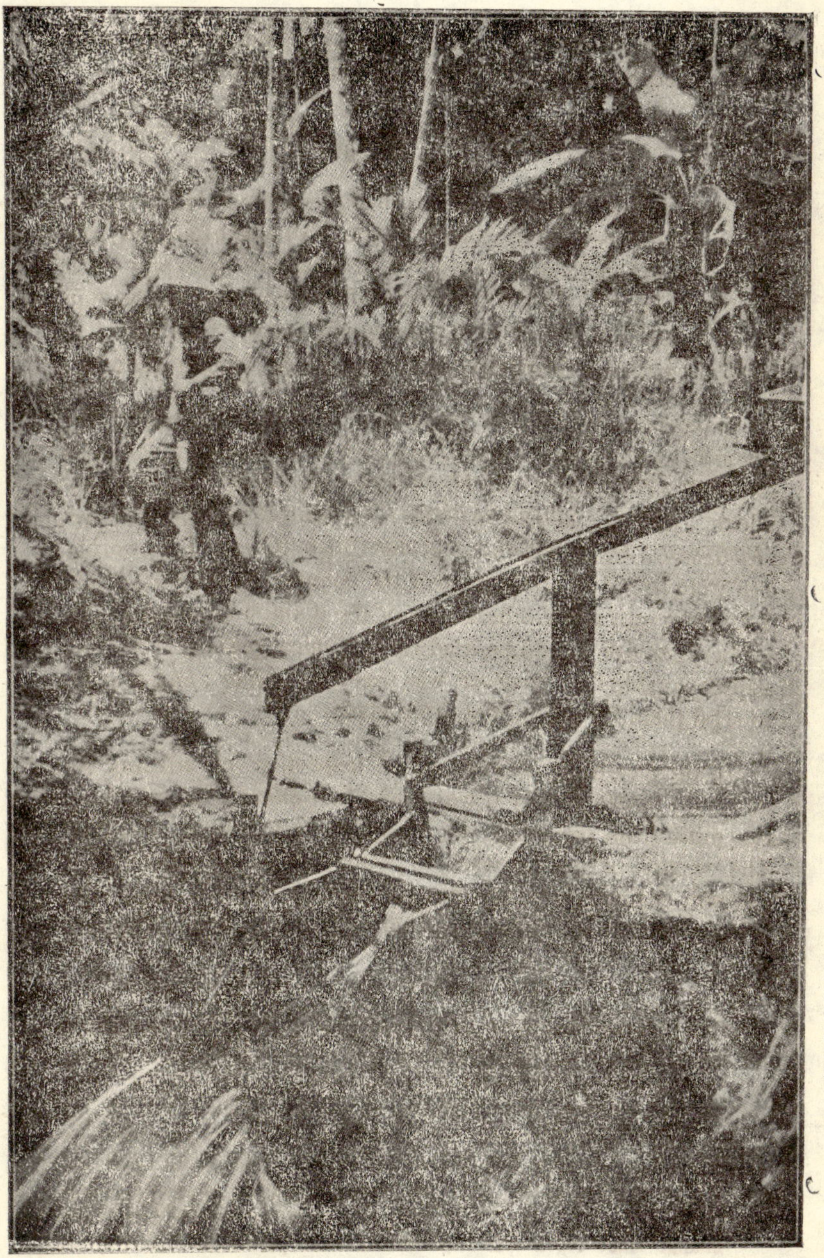

Automatic Flushing Siphon—A Simple Tipping Device
Not used in Yol, Expected to get damaged, Under local conditions.

rocks, passed through the sluice holes, and during heavy rain water overflowed over the damn into the stream.

THE LARVIVOROUS FISH ; SCHIZOTHORAX PROGASTUS

The mosquito breeding in several small streams, ponds, tanks, and *bowlees* continued to be the cause of serious concern. Many of them were used as sources of drinking water by the villagers. The introduction of larvivorous fish was considered the ideal solution. *Gambosia affinis* (top minnow) had been imported in India and was being widely recommended.

Indigenous larvivorous fishes were known. In Sylhet, for example, commonest larvivorous fish reported were : *Barbus phutunia* (*Tith puti*) ; *Nuria daurica* (*Ophicephalus straiatus* Bloch (*upol*) ; *Anabus scarelens* (*Koi*) : *Haplocilus panchux* (*Kampona*) ; *Ophiocephalus punctalus* Boch (*Gorvi*). Larvivorous fish were found in other areas of the country. Baini Prasad and S.L. Hora and a few others were of the opinion that indigenous larvivorous fish should be used for biological reasons.* The readily available fish, however, was *Gambosia affinis* ; and requests to send them for use in Yol, were made.

In the meantime, during routine inspection of streams for mosquito larvae density it was found that along a stream about two miles from the camp no mosquito larvae were breeding. The results of examination of water, its temperature, salt content, chemical composition and flora, etc. didnot differ from other streams with heavy mosquito-larval breeding. The very

*The position regarding larvivorous fishes is discussed in the chapter on "Anti-Larval Measures" of this book. Dr. Baini Prasad, an authority on this subject on the draft of this chapter wrote to the author on December 1, 1944 : "The section in regard to the Larvivorous fish about which alone I can make any suggestions is very well drawn up, and I donot think I can add anything more to it. My views on the subject to use indigenous larvivorous fish instead of imported have not undergone any change since Hora and I published our paper on Larvivorous fishes".

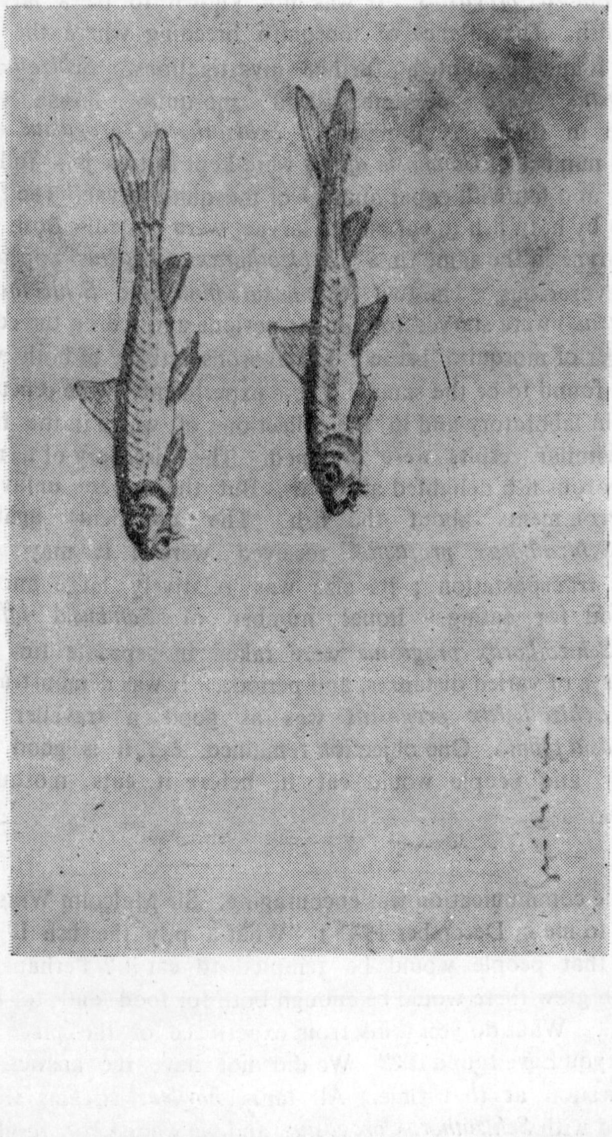

Larvivorous Fish of Yol Schizothorax Progastus

observant and capable malaria inspector Mr. Kher Singh drew my attention to the presence of fish in the stream which was free from larvae. Thus began a series of investigations on *Schizothorax progastus.* It was not known to be a larvivorous fish. The absence of mosquito breeding where the fish was found prompted further investigations. *Schizothorax progastus* were dessected and mosquito larvae were found in them. A number of *Schizorhorax progastus* and equal number of *Gambosia affinis* were kept in two jars full of water and fed with equal number of mosquito larvae. The time taken by both fish to eat all the larvae were noted. Both ate the larvae in the same time ; *Schizothorax progastus* appeared more voracious. The two (*Gambusia affinis* and *Schizothorax progastus*) were starved for similar periods and fed on the equal number of mosquito larvae. Larvivorous activity of both was again found to be the same. These experiments were repeated both in laboratory and in the collections of water in the field and similar results were obtained. The discovery of a new larvivorous fish delighted all of us. But there were unfavourable comments about the fish. The comments against the *Schizothorax prorastus* received were : it may not stand transportation ; its size was relatively large and it is good for eating. Equal number of *Gambusia affinis* and *Schizothorax progastus* were taken in separate tins on journeys of varied distances, and periods. It was demonstrated that *Schizothorax progastus* was as good a traveller as *Gambusia affinis.* One objection remained, *i.e.* it is good for eating and people would eat it, before it eats mosquito larvae.

One communication was encouraging. Sir Malcolm Watson wrote to me in December 1945 : "What a pity the fish is so large that people would be tempted to eat it ? Perhaps if enough grew there would be enough both for food and to kill larvae ? What do you think from experience of the place in which you have found it ?" We did not have the answer to the question at that time. All tanks, *bowlees*, streams were stocked with *Schizothorax progastus*, and we waited for results.

No larvae were found in places where this fish was introduced.*

It can be now stated that the size of *Schizothorax progastus* and its quality of good for eating are not found as barriers to its use as larvivorous fish. The report of Mr. V.N. Rao sent to the author by Lt. Colonel Pillai in 1949, mentioned above states :

"It (*Schizothorax progastus*) is progressing quite well ; their number in big *Bowlees* vary from 75-150, in small ones about 50 ; they are in some parts of streams and in Nod—Khad also ; they (*Bowlees* and streams with *Schizothorax progastus*) are completely free from breeding and experiments were carried out to test their larvicidal qualities as compared with *Gambusia affinis*. The results were quite satisfactory : These fish were also left in several static tanks of the camp with good results. But it is noticed that these fish donot thrive the moment the water gets dirty. It is found this species has been introduced in some *Bowlees* in the Tanda camp near Kangra. They are thriving quite well there too."

DECLINE IN INCIDENCE OF MALARIA

By the end of 1945 there was marked decline in the incidence of malaria. During September 1942 (the peak periods) malaria incidence in the camp was 22 per 1000. In the same month in 1945 it was below 3 per 1000. There were imported cases 118 in 1944 and 67 in 1945. It is difficult to measure the proportion of this decline due to bio-environmental measures taken during 1942-1945, as other malaria control measures were concurrently taken such as malaria discipline regarding clothing, (long sleeve shirts and pants in the evening), use of mosquito nets, observance of weekly Dry Day, antimosquito

*Raina, B.L., *Schizothorax progastus*, *Indian Medical Gazette*, V LXXX 5, p. 273, 1945.

measures, early detection and treatment of malaria cases, along with health education for the strict observance of the recommended measures. But considering the elimination of most of the mosquito breeding places, it may be justifiable to attribute major decline due to bio-environmental measures.

The experience in Yol, further supports the view that the use of indigenous larvivorous fish should be promoted ; they flourish in their natural surroundings, eat the mosquito larvae, without disturbing other useful flora and fauna.

APPENDIX D

A NOTE ON MALARIA IN THE PUNJAB [PRE-PARTITION INDIA] DATED 17.7. 1944 BY DR. BUTT DIRECTOR OF PUBLIC HEALTH PUNJAB

The malaria problem in the Punjab is complicated by a number of factors including chiefly : (*i*) canal irrigation which has considerably raised the level of subsoil water, (*ii*) construction of large embankments to intercept huge discharges along hill sides, (*iii*) river floods following heavy monsoon rainfall, and (*iv*) extensive burrow-pits along the roads. As a result chiefly of these conditions malaria has become endemic in the province.

At intervals of years, widespread epidemics of malaria are liable to occur throughout the north-west India more especially in the districts of the Punjab lying within the Indo-gangetic plain. The disastrous epidemic of malaria which broke out with exceptional severity in 1908 was of such a type. In three months it occasioned over 300,000 deaths amongst a population of approximately 20,000,000 in the Punjab. Such epidemics of a regional character usually develop during years of excessive monsoon rainfall associated with overflow of rivers following a series of years in which rainfall has been in defect. The greater the number of years which elapse since the last epidemic year, the more likely is an epidemic to occur.

Organisation of Anti-Malaria Work

The investigation of malaria in the Punjab is centered at the Punjab Epidemiological Bureau and it consists chiefly of (*i*) forecasting the probable incidence of epidemic malaria, and (*ii*) carrying out of malaria surveys in areas adversely affected by this disease with a view to make suitable recommendations for its control.

Every year in the beginning of September a forecast of the probable prevalence of malaria is issued for the whole province. The method of forecasting is based on the hypothesis that malaria epidemics occur owing to the loss of equilibrium between 'infection' and 'immunity', and involve the consideration of the humidity, spleen rate, epidemic potential and economic factors. The combined conditions favourable to the occurrence of an intense epidemic usually are :

(*i*) Conspicuous excess of July-August rainfall over the normal, or extensive floods.

(*ii*) A relatively high epidemic potential factor—above 60.

(*iii*) A low spleen rate in June.

(*iv*) A famine or relatively high prices during the preceding year.

Such forecasts have been invaluable in forestalling measures to combat epidemics of malaria in this province.

Malaria surveys in 16 out of 29 districts in the Punjab have been undertaken during the last five years and the recommendations thus made have been intensively carried out by the district health staff. In this connection it may be pointed out that anti-malaria work in this province has been reorganised with the object of establishing in each district a nucleus of anti-malaria organisation sufficient for the execution of useful routine work and capable of expansion, should malaria assume epidemic proportions. In this manner, each district has been provided with anti-mosquito equipment including pneumatic sprayers, Malariol, Paris green and pyrethrum extract for the destruction of adult anophelines in their day-time resting places.

In addition to the district health staff, a central Field Epidemiological Unit has been functioning since 1939 and undertakes the investigation and control of malaria in different parts of the Punjab. Amongst its personnel are included a highly qualified and experienced Entomologist, two Sub-Assistant Health Officers, one Laboratory Assistant, six Sanitary Supervisors and twelve Sanitary Patrols. In addition to the routine measures which form part of anti-malaria campaigns in the Punjab, the resources of the health department have been mobilised from time to time in dealing with severe outbreaks of malaria. Such a contingency arose in 1942 when this province experienced an exceptionally severe epidemic of regional malaria. The details of the measures undertaken during this epidemic are embodied in the "Review of Health Conditions and Public Health Work in the Punjab during the year 1942".

Only three species of anopheline mosquitoes namely *A. culicifacies*, *A. stephensi* and *A. fluviatilis* are known to transmit malaria in the Punjab. In addition, *A. maculatus*, which is found in large numbers in the vicinity of the foot-hills, has been mentioned as a carrier of malaria but direct evidence to this effect is not available. Of the species mentioned above, *Anopheles culicifacies* is considered to be the chief carrier of malaria in the Punjab.

Systematic records of spleen rate in different districts of the Punjab during 1943 are given below :

Statement Showing the Spleen Rate by Districts in the Punjab for November, 1943

Sr. No.	District	Spleen Rate
1.	Hissar	27.78
2.	Rohtak	22.51
3.	Gurgaon	13.53
4.	Karnal	24.24
5.	Ambala	15.03
6.	Simla	3.35
7.	Kangra	14.48
8.	Hoshiarpur	8.31
9.	Jullundur	5.41

10.	Ludhiana	9.76
11.	Ferozepur	7.57
12.	Lahore	10.94
13.	Amritsar	5.33
14.	Gurdaspur	11.44
15.	Sialkot	8.02
16.	Gujranwala	29.78
17.	Sheikhupura	21.89
18.	Gujrat	11.49
19.	Shahpur	13.64
20.	Jhelum	15.10
21.	Rawalpindi	4.08
22.	Attock	13.58
23.	Mianwali	15.30
24.	Montgomery	11.18
25.	Lyallpur	10.41
26.	Jhang	24.96
27.	Multan	8.36
28.	Muzaffargarh	25.70
29.	Dera Ghazi Khan	5.95
	Provincial Spleen Rate	*13.63*

Malaria Cases

The following figures refer to the total number of malaria cases treated at hospitals and dispensaries in the Punjab during the period from 1933 to 1942, and the incidence of malaria rate which has been calculated on the available figures per 1,000 of the population of the province of the same period :—

Year	No. of malaria cases treated	Incidence of malaria rate
1933	3062837	124.19
1934	2174764	87.78
1935	1846147	73.51
1936	1994392	77.76
1937	1568000	59.93
1938	1494267	55.99
1939	1673530	61.46
1940	2736899	98.60
1941	2898089	101.55
1942	3781172	130.22

From the above data it is evident that the maximum number of malaria cases were treated in 1942 and the incidence of malaria rate was also highest in the same year. Localised epidemics of moderate intensity were experienced in 1933 and 1941.

Deaths due to Malaria

Precise information regarding mortality due to malaria is not available as in most cases the deaths due to this disease are included amongst 'Fever deaths'. The deaths due to fever and figures pertaining to infant mortality during 1933-42 are tabulated below :—

Year	Fever deaths	Fever death-rate	Infant mortality rate
1933	460737	18.68	192.55
1934	461328	18.62	187.40
1935	396328	15.78	155.19
1936	374833	14.61	158.44
1937	376809	14.40	163.04
1938	410198	17.42	166.84
1939	408676	15.01	167.57
1940	473641	17.06	178.22
1941	528635	18.52	185.20
1942	651259	22.08	213.84

The above statistics also suggest the extreme severity of malaria epidemic during 1942 when the fever death rate and infant mortality were excessive.

APPENDIX E

EXTRACTS CIRCULARS DIRECTOR PUBLIC HEALTH

PUBLIC HEALTH DEPARTMENT
CENTRAL PROVINCES AND BERAR
Lt. Col. S.N. MAKAND, IMS

I. Anti-Malarial Measures 4 August 1937

These should aim at :—

(1) Prevention and destruction of mosquito larvae.

(2) Prevention and destruction of adult mosquitoes.

(3) Personal prophylaxis.

(1) Mosquitoes breed in water on surface of which they lay their eggs. In warm countries, eggs hatch out in two or three days and from it a worm-like creature, called a larvae emerges, which lives in water and swims about freely and feeds greedily on minute particles of vegetable and animal matter, both dead and alive. The larvae of malaria-carrying mosquitoes feed at the surface of water and have to come up every now and then to breathe air.

Most mosquitoes prefer fresh, still or stagnant and clean water for breeding, but a few varieties will breed in running water and some in dirty or salt water. Most mosquitoes require sheltered and shady or partially shady places for breeding. This is afforded by weeds, grasses, bushes, etc., growing on the margin of ponds, streams, nullahs, etc. Some mosquitoes, however, prefer breeding in places exposed to sunshine. Removal of weeds, grasses and other vegetation from potential breeding places is, however, necessary to promote evaporation and drying up of collection of water, to bring to light breeding places which might be overlooked and to facilitate application of anti-larval measures. Mosquitoes prefer small pools and collections of water and the margins and shallow portions of large sheets of water, where they can obtain protection from winds and currents and where they can obtain sufficiency of food materials.

The varying habits of different species of mosquitoes indicate the necessity of carefully studying the prevailing type of malaria-carrying mosquitoes in any particular locality in order to deal effectively with them. What may be successful in one case may have the contrary effect in another.

The larvae feeds and grows for about 6 or 7 days and then it changes its shape and becomes inactive, but has to come up to the surface to breathe. In this stage it is called a "pupa". After one or two days the skin of the pupa splits and a fully-formed mosquito comes out and flies away.

Under favourable conditions, in warm climate, the cycle of development of the mosquito inside water takes about 7—10 days. This is important to know as it indicates that anti-larval measures in connection with collections of water, in which mosquitoes are apt to breed. must be applied and *repeated once every week*. If longer intervals are allowed, many mosquitoes will complete their period of development and escape to feed on human beings and carry malaria.

From a knowledge of the breeding habits of mosquitoes it is obvious that the most radical method of preventing mosquitoes is to deny them facilities for breeding and to destroy them while they are yet in water. This can be accomplished by eliminating all collections of water near and around human habitations and to deal with unavoidable collections in such a manner as to render them inaccessible to mosquitoes or unsuitable for their breeding or to destroy mosquito larvae wherever they find opportunities to form.

Action to be taken, therefore, consist of :—

Prevention of collections of water in and around human

habitations—(1) Small collections, as in broken bottles, crockery and *gharas*, in empty tins, etc., are fruitful sources of mosquitoes. These should not be thrown about but broken up and buried. Gutters and drains should be regularly cleaned to prevent their being clogged up, leading to accumulation of fluids. Garden tanks and sumps, fire buckets, branch irrigation channels, etc., should be cleaned out and completely emptied or treated with anti-larval oils once a week. Receptacles such as *gharas*, buckets, pots, etc., should not be left lying about neglected. If not regularly used, they should be placed upside down so as not to collect rain water.

Excavations for earth, stones, "moorum", etc., and brick-fields should not be allowed within a mile of the periphery of a town or village. In determining sites for such operations, due consideration should be paid to the possibilities of future extension and expansion of such places.

In the construction of roads, embankments, etc., care should be taken to provide adequate outlets for the natural drainage of the area.

Roadsides excavations for earth or "moorum", for the dressing of the surface and sides of roads, should be so made as to obtain continuous and properly-graded channels which will serve to drain away rain water, instead of allowing it to accumulate in pools and ditches.

(2) Small depressions and pits, pot holes, etc., should be filled up with refuse, earth and debris. Holes in tree trunks and large branches should be filled up with stones and mud.

(3) Water cisterns and wells, particularly disused wells, should be provided with gauze or other cover to prevent access of mosquitoes. Disused wells or those which are very little used are favourable breeding places for mosquitoes. Wells, used for drinking, cannot be oiled but may be treated with Petrol (about one ounce for $3\frac{1}{2}$ square feet of water surface), which kills the larvae almost immediately. It should be applied in the evening. In two or three hours the smell and taste of petrol disappears.

The best method is to stock wells with larvae-eating fish.

Clean powdered cork has been recommended for wells. The powder is thrown over the water surface where it floats and prevents mosquitoes from laying eggs and suffocates the larvae.

(4) Waste water from wells is often found teeming with mosquito larvae. The waste water should be thoroughly drained away or collected in sharply-defined pits or trenches, which should be treated with larvicide once a week. To prevent overflow, the pits should be partially evacuated now and then and the liquid used for watering roads and gardens or spread over plots of land in the vicinity. Prevention of bathing and washing of clothes and utensils at or near wells will help in greatly reducing the amount of waste water and will help in keeping down mosquitoes.

(5) Edges of large collections of water, which cannot be drained or eliminated by filling, such as large tanks should be trimmed and kept steep and free from vegetation and accumulation of debris. If possible, the edges should be paved or stone-pitched. Edges, where mosquitoes are likely to breed or where larvae are seen, should be treated with anti-larval oils once a week.

Streams should be properly canalized by having their sides sloped at an angle of about 45° in order to obtain an even and swift flow of water. Embankments should be lined with large stones and vegetation cleared from the edges. Pools left after the overflow of the stream during rains should be drained back into the stream.

(6) Drains should be as narrow as possible, in proportion to the amount of water they have to carry, and should be given an adequate fall. This will secure self-cleansing action and prevent stagnation. The sides of the drain should be sloped at an angle of 50° to 60°. The sides, edges and the bed should be kept free from vegetation.

Drains should be cleaned regularly. In case of *kuccha*

drains, at least once weekly removal of deposited silt and sludge is necessary to maintain a free flow of its contents.

Larvae-eating fish. Stocking of wells, tanks, tanks and ponds with such fish will diminish the number of mosquitoes. The best fish for this purpose is Gambusia affinis (See Circular No. 539, dated the 21st January 1937). Other useful varieties are :—

> *Haplochilus lineolatus* ("Piku") and *Anabas scandens* ("Khajura"). One dozen "Khajuras" are sufficient for fifteen square feet of water surface.

II. The Control of Mosquito Breeding by Herbage Packing 29 November 1938

Freshly cut green herbage (stems up to a finger breadth in diameter with leaves attached) is laid in the beds of streams or drains. The stems are laid with their butts pointing upstream to avoid obstruction to the flow of water. The herbage is well trampled underfoot, and packed so as to form a dense cover 2 or 3 feet deep. Fallen trees, boulders, etc., should be removed from the channel as far as possible before packing. If there is a considerable current, the lower end of the packed section should be provided with a double row of stakes or other form of fencing, to prevent dislocation of the herbage.

The object of the method is to alter the composition of the water, thus making it unsuitable for malaria-carrying mosquitoes, which almost invariably require clear, fresh water to breed in. Hence the necessity of using fresh green herbage which will rot readily. Culicine mosquitoes breed freely in water charged with organic matter, so that the method is unsuitable where it is necessary to combat a general mosquito nuisance.

Herbage packing is specially applicable in foot-hill regions where the dangerous malaria carriers breed in streams and drains during the period immediately preceding the rains. The packing is of course washed away when the heavy rains commence, but by that time the stream is harmless as a source of mosquito breeding.

III. The Use of Oil Booms as an Anti-mosquito Measure 15 February 1939

———

The object of oil booms is the destruction of mosquito larvae in moving water whether these are produced by local breeding, or are being carried into the area to be controlled from upstream (larval drift). The booms are placed at varying intervals, which can only be determined by actual experience. The most important is that which is placed at the upper end of the controlled section of the channel. The type of boom to be employed depends on various circumstances, such as the width of the channel, the velocity of the current, the amount of water present at different times, whether the channel is used by boats, etc. In the last named case, it is of course impossible to use a boom which traverses the whole width of the channel.

The following types of boom have been found effective in Delhi :—

(1) In small drains and irrgation channels where the current is never very strong booms made from *sarkanda* (*moonj*) grass were placed across the whole width of the channel, and fixed to vertical stakes, the lower edge of the boom being several inches above the bed. The *sarkanda* grass was fixed with its stems parallel with the surface of the water, the object being to trap the larvae without seriously impeding the flow of water. *Bhoosa* (chaff), soaked in oil containing 2½ per cent cresol, was thrown on to the surface of the water above the boom, so that the larvae trapped by the latter were destroyed by the oil exuding from the *bhoosa*. This procedure leads to economy in oil, which is otherwise rapidly carried away downstream.

(2) In the case of a canal distributory, 22 feet wide, it was necessary to devise a boom which would operate when the canal was running full, and also when the flow as reduced to a depth of a few inches by the periodical cutting off of the supply higher up. The boom consisted of three sections, each made of

sarkanda grass in the form of a *chick*, which could be rolled up when required. When the water was low, only the central section was used, whilst when the canal was full, all three sections were brought into use, being rolled up from the bottom to the desired height. The boom was supported by wooden stakes driven into the bed of the canal, and *bhoosa* soaked in oil was thrown on to the water above the boom as in (1) above.

(3) In the case of a large drain which had a number of slight curves in its course, it was observed that mosquito larvae were not uniformly distribured along it, but tended to congregate at certain definite spots. Short booms, projecting only a few feet from the banks, were placed at these spots, oil-soaked *bhoosa* being thrown on to the water above each boom.

It is usually necessary to have some sort of arrangement for holding up objects which may float down the stream and damage the booms. A single rope stretched across from bank to bank is quite effective for this purpose.

All oil-booms need a good deal of attention, and in every section where they are used some one has to be constantly on the watch to prevent people from tampering with them. But their use leads to economy in oil and they probably constitute the most effective method of dealing with the difficult problem of larval drift.

It should be emphasized that all the types of booms described above are still in the experimental stage and will probably need to be modified to suit local conditions.

APPENDIX F

EXTRACTS FROM MALARIA IN SIND [Pre-partition]

By

Dr. B.J. Ajwani, Malariologist, Government of Sind

General

The area of the province of Sind is 47,000 square miles. The population according to the 1941 Census is 45,35,000. Eighty per cent of the population, that is to say 36,40,315 inhabitants live in villages. The main occupation of the country people is agriculture. Sind depends on the water supply of the river Indus to which it owes its life. The land is cultivated by irrigation whose importance from the point of view of Malaria is great. The extent of land irrigated in Sind in the year 1940-41 was 60,70,410 acres.

Previous Survey

The Sind Malaria Enquiry Committee commenced its work in the year 1927 when preliminary investigations were undertaken by Lieut-Col. T.C. Mc Combie Young, I.M.S., and Jamadar Abdul Majid, I.M.D., who carried out field surveys in the Upper Sind Frontier, Sukkur and Larkana Districts in Northern Sind. Their report included an analysis of the taluka epidemic figures for the whole of the Province and a discussion as to the probable effects of the Llyod Barrage Project on the incidence of Malaria.

From May 1928 until May 1935, Rai Saheb J.D. Baily, I.M.D., was in charge of the field work under the general direction of Lieut-Col. G. Covell, I.M.S., Systematic Malaria Surveys were undertaken in selected areas in all the talukas of

Sind which were to come under the operation of the Barrage Scheme, and also in certain tracts lying outside this area.

(1) Before the Llyod Barrage Scheme commmenced operations, many parts of Sind were highly malarious and the province was subject to periodical epidemics of malaria, more especially affecting the northern areas. The contention put forward in certain quarters that most, if not all, of the malaria now existing in Sind is due to the operation of the Barrage Scheme is thus unsupported by facts.

(2) Nevertheless it is a fact that malarial conditions in Sind have become considerably worse since the Barrage Scheme began to operate, and we consider that this is due mainly to conditions favouring the spread of malaria brought about by the operation of the scheme.

(3) The principal factors which have produced this adverse effect are :—

(*i*) a rise in the subsoil water level in many areas ;

(*ii*) actual or threatened water-logging of the soil in certain areas ;

(*iii*) seepage from some of the new canals ;

(*iv*) the cutting off of sections of certain of the old canals, thus forming prolific anopheline breeding grounds ;

(*v*) the formation of the 'lake' above the Barrage with a corresponding rise of the subsoil water level along the course of the Indus ; and

(*vi*) an extension in rice cultivation in areas outside the Barrage command in northern Sind due to the increased supply of water made available by the presence of the Barrage lake and the re-modelling of pre-existing canals.

(4) The future course of events as regards the incidence of malaria depends on the degree of success attained by the irriga-

tion Department in providing efficient drainage and preventing the evils of water logging.

(5) It is strongly urged that increased facilities for the treatment of malaria be provided throughout the area affected by the Barrage Scheme.

(6) We also recommend that where possible all rest houses provided for officials touring in Sind be rendered mosquito proof, equipped with electric lights and fans.

(7) Attention is drawn to the vital importance of making a soil and sub-soil survey of the area involved as well as providing efficient scheme of drainage before any large irrigation project is undertaken.

Malaria Problem of Sind

From the results of limited surveys done in Sukkur, Larkana and Thar Parkar Districts, it is seen that malaria has increased after the construction of the Lloyd Barrage and Canal Construction as judged by the increase in dispensary statistics and spleen rates. On account of increased supply of water due to the creation of Barrage Lake, great extension of rice cultivation, rise in the sub-soil water level, cutting off the loops of old canals in which water is still stagnating as Ghar Canal, and Old Sukkur Canal, and perennial canals which supply water through out the year thus affecting the drainage capacity of the soil. In Bechanji some fruit gardens were ruined on account of rise of subsoil water and in other places dry cultivation has given place to rice cultivation and Puban cultivation. Sinton remarks "Unfortunately in connection with certain other irrigation schemes initiated in recent years, the results of experience gained in the past, and repeated warnings, have passed apparently unheeded, or imperfect measures have been carried out, with the result that the harmful effects are already being felt and it is practically certain that these may be disastrus in future to large areas (Sind)". The subsoil water levels at Dokri show that in the month of October water rises by about 4 feet in Dry area and by 6 feet in Wet area.

Year	Dry Area		Wet Area	
	Maximum	Minimum	Maximum	Minimum
1939-40	4.7 (7.10.39)	9.1 (16.5.40)	1.91 (1.10.39)	7.96 (1.6.40)
1940-41	4.2 (1.10.40)	8.95 (15.6.40)	1.80 (15.9.40)	7.82 (1.5.40)

"Malarial trouble continued throughout the year resulting in death of labour specially during the month of November and December", (Director of Agricuture 1940-41).

At the 12th Conference of the Medical Research Workers in 1934, Resolution No. 11 reads :—

"This conference notes the rise of malaria that has occurred as the result of the Sind Irrigation Project and regrets that the definite early warnings of the Malaria Survey in this respect had apparently gone unheeded".

Malaria is the heavy burden that Sind is carrying on its weak shoulders. It cause 70 deaths daily directly and 35 indirectly due to deaths from phthisis. dysentery, diarrhoea, and pneumonia. The economic loss sustained by each individual as calculated by Russell in one of the villages in Madras is Rs. 3-14-0 per capita per year for treatment of malaria and loss of wages. Here is direct loss of the people of Sind of about Rs. 1,60,00,000.

Three Problems of Rural Malaria

(*i*) Rice Cultivation.

(*ii*) Irrigation Malaria.

(*iii*) Epidemic Malaria.

Preventive Measures

(1) Drainage scheme on the right bank of the Indus river. Efficient drainage should be provided for the surplus water on

the right bank. In any town where pipe water supply is introduced it is preceded by a drainage system.

(2) Intermittent Irrigation by which is meant periodical withholding of water just long enough to permit the surface of fields and channels to become sufficiently dry to cause the death of all mosquito larvae is tried in South India, where the land is dried for 2-2½ days. This method should be introduced in Sind.

Similar experiment of intermittent irrigation should be performed in Larkana taluka.

(3) Rice cultivation should only be permitted where it was cultivated in the pre-barrage days. On account of the "Grow More Food" policy, it is intended to extend rice cultivation in Sind. Any extension of rice cultivation in Sind will be suicidal to the health of the people.

Rice cultivation should be prohibited within 2 miles radious of large towns and 1 mile radious of small towns. On that land vegetables should be cultivated by lift by means of Persian Wheels on the wells. I have seen that wherever vegetables are cultivated by this method near the town, malaria is less (Khanpur-Sukkur District). Vegetables pay more than rice crop but the cultivation of vegetables requires hard labour while rice is known to be "Lazy man's Crop".

Irrigation Malaria

In the perennial irrgation water is carried by the canals which are constructed at high levels so that water is supplied to the fields by gravity. The main canals and the large branches do not breed mosquitoes so long they are running full. The numerous borrow pits by the sides of the canals, residual pools in the bed of the canals when they are emptied, afford opportunity for the breeding of dangerous mosquitoes. All the fields channels which are prolific source of *A. culicifacies* should be under the supervision and control of the Public Works Department authorities and weeds should be regularly removed, their sides trained and leakage stopped. Several Zamindars have their own water channels run parallel to one another in the same place. Most of the larvae die if water is allowed to flow in each channel for seven days and kept dry for seven days. I often noticed that the roadside channels contain water though they are seldom used for road watering. Water should be allowed alternately in the road channels and when it is required.

(2) *Water logging.* The seepage water from Rohri Canal in Khairpur State and from Dadu and Rice Canals near Larkana should be stopped.

(3) The existing pits near the villages and burrow pits along the canals and roads should be filled in by obtaining the earth from

(*a*) high lands in shallow and their slices.

(*b*) from the bed of the canals.

No more burrow pits should be allowed along the railway line, roads and canals.

(4) Water channels should not be allowed to flow through the towns.

(5) Loops of old canals should be filled in with refuse.

(6) Pabun cultivation should not be allowed near the towns.

APPENDIX G

EXTRACT FROM THE REPORT OF DR. C.N. SHUKLA MEDICAL OFFICER

NAWAPARA DATED 20.2.44

Paddy-fields. These are particularly dangerous when the paddy plant is less than one foot high, as at this stage they breed the carrier species. When plants attain a height of more than one foot, the carrier species cease to breed and their place is taken up by other species which prefer some shade for the development of larvae. As fields are not artificially irrigated, observance of a dry day or intermittent irrigation are out of question. What we can do is to stop further addition of fields within a radius of one mile from the village. No new fields should be created within this limit and those that are lying uncultivated and with bunds should be drained out so that there will be no accumulation of rain-water in them.

In hilly regions, the mistake has been made of selecting sites immediately along-side streams which are the chief sources of breading of the carrier species. Almost all villages in this range face a stream. If the stream lies at some distance from the village, trees should be planted thickly in between the stream and village, so that they may act as a barrier against the infiltration of mosquitoes. If there is a belt of forest intervening the village and the stream, it should on no account be either thinned or cut. In choosing the site for new establishment of a village, it is advisible to select a position which is remote from anopheline breeding places. As it is the mosquito which has fed on an infected human being that is dangerous, it is advisible to select a site which is as far a possible away from a malarious village. This precaution should always be exercised during the construction of Dak Bungalows.

These should be kept free of vegetations as they afford a shelter to larvae against equatic, enemies, give them partial shade against the hot sun and supply them with food. If possible a barrier of tall trees should always be planted between a village and tank. *Trapa bispinosa* or water-nut plant (*Singhara*) is said to inhibit larval development and should be planted in tanks.

Zoo-prophylaxis. Animal prophylaxis against malaria, though not an important measure of control may reduce the number of mosquito-bites. Two of the three carrier species here are usually found in cattle sheds also and prefer bovine blood along with human blood. Cattle-sheds should always be located on the outskirts of a village instead of indiscriminately as is usually the case, between the breeding places and the village. This will make the inhabitants more free from the attack of mosquitoes as most of the mosquitoes may satisfy their hunger on cattle-blood first.

Cultivation of alleged deterrent trees and plants. Experiments have proved that trees so far used have no direct effect against adult mosquitoes. The planting has a good effect by drawing up water and reducing the level of sub-soil water. Trees recommended are Casuarine, Nim, Eucalyptus, Cauna, Sun-flower, Castor-oil plant. etc.

Precautionary mesaures during the construction of roads and buildings. Mosquitoes require water in which to breed but they exhibit very definite preferences in selection of their breeding places. Malaria-carrying mosquitoes do not ordinarily breed in filthy water. Many of the breeding places have resulted from man-made conditions. In malaria-control the chief object therefore is to prevent accumulation of useless water and to manipulate it in an intelligent manner.

Excavation of earth from burrow-pits is a most dangerous and universal practice. For repairs of roads and for various other purposes, earth is excavated in such a way as depressions are left behind and collect water specially in rains. The only out-let of this water is soakage into the ground. On both sides of roads chains of burrow-pits are formed extending for miles together. These hold water for a sufficiently long time, to allow a complete life-cycle of mosquitoes. This leaves behind a lasting source of trouble which is to be dealt with by expensive filling operations if funds ever permit and for this reason, it is very essential that every precaution should be exercised during the time of construction when many of the evils can be prevented at little or no additional cost. The essential thing is to obviate earth removal in any way which will lead to subsequent retention of water. The removal of earth so as to leave behind a continuous line of excavation in the form of a drain may serve the purpose. As the range of flight of anopheles is not usually more than a mile, it is necessary not to make burrow-pits within a mile of villages. It is always preferable to spend a little more money in the beginning, in getting earth from a higher ground, perhaps involving a little longer load than to take earth from already existing burrow-pits nearer the road and involving shorter load. A little extra amount thus spent will in many cases be more than compensated by the prevention of malaria in the locality. The drain if constructed will supply earth and morrum and also carry storm-water during rains. If at all earth or morrum is badly needed and finances are limited, the existing pits should be further deepened but on no account be made wider. This does not increase the surface area of a breeding place.

Similarly while constructing culverts ; the formation of a pool at the out-fall end due to excavation of earth should always be borne in mind and the area should be rammed with stones with a thin plaster of cement above, if possible.

Dak Bungalows and inspection huts. A large number of Inspection huts have been provided for inspecting officers. Though it is a known fact that the whole of the range is a malarious one, mosquito-screening in such bungalows has not been provided. Money utilised in construction of new bungalows can be well utilised in screening the present ones. With the development of rapid motor transport facilities it would not be necessary to screen every Dak Bungalow ; even if one Dak Bungalow in every 20 mile length is properly screened to begin with, it will serve a useful purpose. As anopheles usually carry on their blood-sucking operations in the dusk and at night ; it would form economic consideration, be sufficient at first to screen the doors, windows and varandahs or only bed and dining rooms which are used at night. The wire gauze recommended for screening should be of 14 mesh and of 30 S.W.G. wire giving an aperture of about 0.055 to 0.057 inch.

APPENDIX H

CHILD HEALTH INFORMATION ON MALARIA

"*Facts for Life** is a practical contribution to the evolving primary health care movement. Intended principally for the developing world, its national and international versions bring togather today's essential family information on maternal and child health care. That information—about birth-spacing, safe motherhood, breast feeding, weaning and child growth, immunization, diarrhoeal diseases, respiratory infections, domestic hygiene, malaria and AIDS—could now enable most families in developing world to make significant improvements in their own and their children's health. *Facts for Life* is therefore an aid to achieving the first level of primary health care—a well informed community".

"*Facts for Life* is a challenge to communicators of all kinds —politicians, educators, religious leaders, health professionals, business leaders, trade unions, voluntary organizations and the mass media. It is for all those who can help to make the contents part of every family's basic stock of child-care Knowledge".

**Facts for Life*, UNICEF, New Delhi, 1991.

The Unique and valuable book Facts for Life "published by UNICEF, WHO and UNESCO in portnership with many of the world's leading medical and children organization", is devised and produced for UNICEF, WHO and UNESCO by P & LA, 18 Observatory Close, Bensen Oxfordshire, OX9 6NU, U.K., Indian Edition is published by UNICEF India Country Office New Delhi printed by Mayar Printers in January, 1990. Two copies are available on request from UNICEF Information Services 73 Lodi Estate, New Delhi 110003.

On "What every family and community has a right to know about malaria, it underlines that : In areas where malaria is common, all families and communities should have access to today's information on preventing and treating the disease".

The six prime health messages could help to prevent the tragedy of over a million* malaria cases each year in India, causing many of child deaths and many more cases of child malnutrition.

"Communicators should also be aware that the effective prevention of malaria depends upon community action and government support".

The six Malaria-Prime Messages are :

"1. Young children should be protected from mosquito bites, especially at night.

2. Communities should destroy mosquito larvae and prevent mosquitoes from breeding.

3. Wherever malaria is common, pregnant women should take anti-malaria tablets throughout pregnancy.

4. Wherever malaria is common, a child who has a fever should be taken to a health worker. If malaria appears to be the cause, the child should be given a full course of an anti-malaria drug.

5. A child with a fever should be kept cool but not cold.

6. A child recovering from malaria needs plenty of liquids and food".

The communicator can further explain that :

*Positive cases of malaria in India reported in 1987 (provisional) were 1.663,284 ; with 185 deaths.

"1. Young children should be protected from mosquito bites, especially at night.

Malaria is spread by the bite of a mosquito. Care should be taken to keep mosquitoes away from young children. There are several ways of doing this :—

By using mosquito nets (preferably impregnated with a mosquito repellent).

By using fumigants such as mosquito coils.

By putting screens on house windows and doors.

By killing mosquitoes in the house.

All members of the community should be protected against mosquito bites. A mosquito can take malaria from an infected person and pass it on to someone who is uninfected.

2. Communities should destroy mosquito larvae and prevent mosquitoes from breeding.

Mosquitoes breed wherever stagnant water can collect : in ponds, swamps, pools, pits, drains, sometimes even tin cans and hoof-prints. They may also breed along the edges of streams. Filling in or draining places where water collects, or spreading oil on ponds and swamps, can kill the mosquito larvae.

Regular clean-ups of the neighbourhood help reduce mos-quto breeding.

3 Wherever malaria is common, pregnant women should take anti-malaria tablets throughout pregnancy.

Pregnant women are more than twice as likely to suffer from malaria. The disease is also more dangerous during pregnancy. It can lead to severe anaemia ('thin blood'), and may cause a miscarriage, premature birth, or still-birth. Babies born to women with malaria are also very likely to be small, weak, and vulnerable to infections.

Pregnant women can be effectively protected against malaria by taking anti-malaria tablets regularly throughout pregnancy.

Anti-malaria tablets should be obtained from a clinic or health workers as not all anti-malarials are safe to take during pregnancy.

4. Wherever malaria is common, a child who has a fever should be taken to a health worker. If malaria appears to be the cause, the child should be given a full course of an anti-malaria drug.

A child with a fever, believed to be caused by malaria, should be given a course of anti-malaria tablets. This course may last between one and ten days (young babies may be given an anti-malaria syrup).

A child should be given the full course of treatment, even if the fever disappears rapidly.

Even if malaria is common, unaffected children should not take anti-malaria tablets every day, as this may prevent the child from building up a natural resistance to malaria.

5. A child with a fever should be kept cool but not cold.

Children with fever should be kept cool by :—

Giving a temperature-reducing medicine (such as paracetamol).

Sponging or bathing with cool (not cold) water.

Not putting too many clothes or blankets on the child.

6. A child recovering from malaria needs plenty of liquids and food.

Malaria burns up energy and the child loses a lot of liquid through sweating. As soon as the child can take food and drink again, these losses should be replaced. Plenty of food and liquid, when the child is recovering from malaria, will help to prevent malnutrition and dehydration".

Index

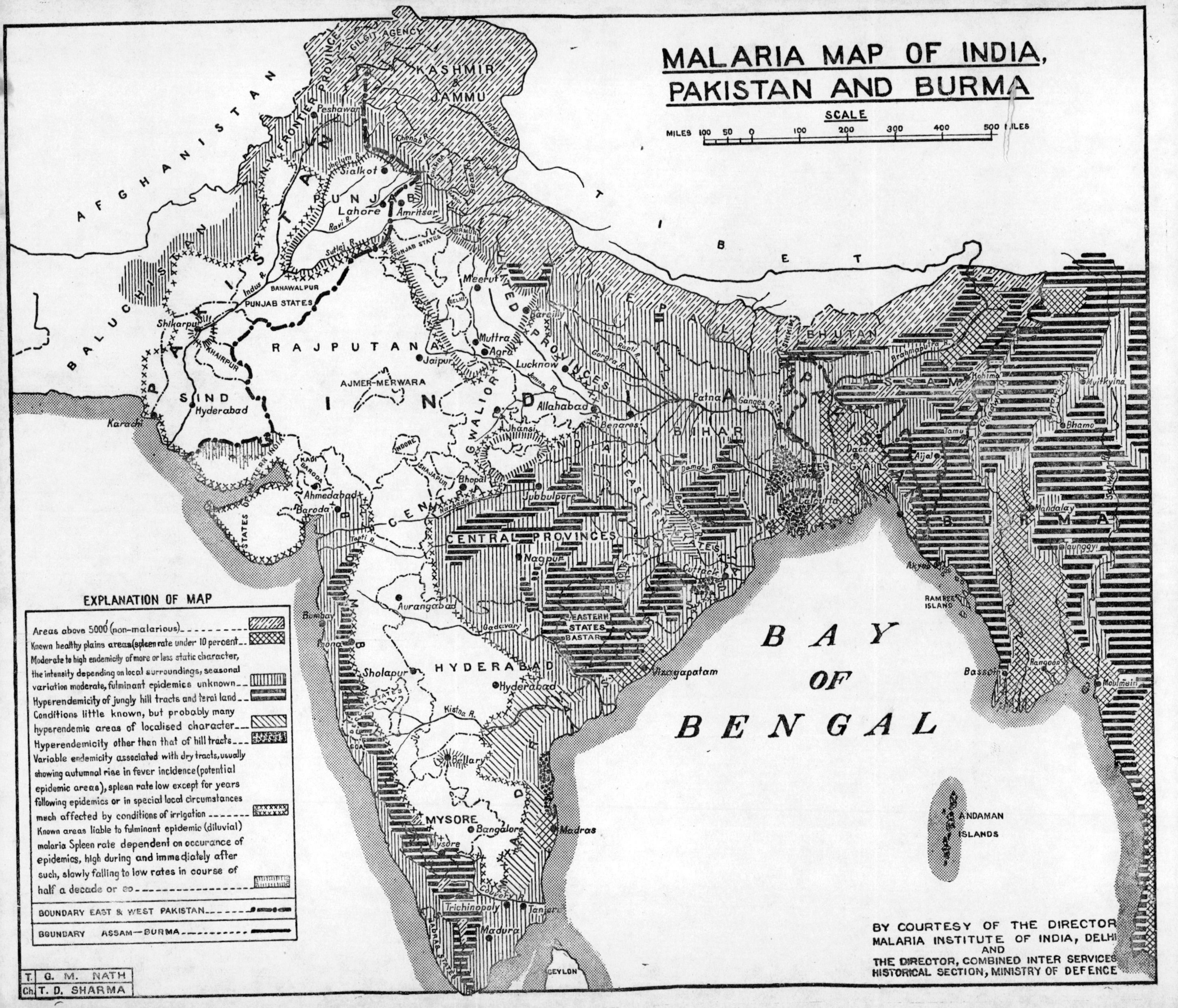
MALARIA MAP OF INDIA, PAKISTAN AND BURMA
SCALE
MILES 100 50 0 100 200 300 400 500 MILES
EXPLANATION OF MAP
Areas above 5000' (non-malarious)
Known healthy plains areas (spleen rate under 10 percent
Moderate to high endemicity of more or less static character, the intensity depending on local surroundings, seasonal variation moderate, fulminant epidemics unknown
Hyperendemicity of jungly hill tracts and terai land
Conditions little known, but probably many hyperendemic areas of localised character
Hyperendemicity other then that of hill tracts
Variable endemicity associated with dry tracts, usually showing autumnal rise in fever incidence (potential epidemic areas), spleen rate low except for years following epidemics or in special local circumstances much affected by conditions of irrigation
Known areas liable to fulminant epidemic (diluvial) malaria Spleen rate dependent on occurance of epidemics, high during and immediately after such, slowly falling to low rates in course of half a decade or so
BOUNDARY EAST & WEST PAKISTAN
BOUNDARY ASSAM—BURMA
AFGHANISTAN
BALUCHISTAN
PAKISTAN
TIBET
KASHMIR & JAMMU
GILGIT AGENCY
PUNJAB
RAJPUTANA
SIND
INDIA
NEPAL
BHUTAN
ASSAM
BIHAR
BENGAL
UNITED PROVINCES
CENTRAL PROVINCES
CENTRAL INDIA
EASTERN STATES
HYDERABAD
MYSORE
MADRAS
BURMA
BAY OF BENGAL
ANDAMAN ISLANDS
CEYLON
Peshawar
Sialkot
Lahore
Amritsar
Meerut
Delhi
Bareilly
Muttra
Agra
Jaipur
Lucknow
Allahabad
Benares
Patna
Jhansi
Karachi
Hyderabad
Shikarpur
Ahmedabad
Baroda
Bhopal
Jubbulpore
Nagpur
Calcutta
Dacca
Cuttack
Aurangabad
Bombay
Poona
Sholapur
Bellary
Bangalore
Mysore
Madras
Trichinopoly
Tanjore
Madura
Vizagapatam
Mandalay
Bhamo
Myitkyina
Kohima
Rangoon
Bassein
Moulmein
BY COURTESY OF THE DIRECTOR
MALARIA INSTITUTE OF INDIA, DELHI
AND
THE DIRECTOR, COMBINED INTER SERVICES
HISTORICAL SECTION, MINISTRY OF DEFENCE
T. G. M. NATH
Ch. T. D. SHARMA